THE Clean20

Also by Ian K. Smith, M.D.

Nonfiction

Blast the Sugar Out!

The SHRED Power Cleanse

The SHRED Diet Cookbook

SUPER SHRED

SHRED

The Truth About Men

Eat

Happy

The 4 Day Diet

Extreme Fat Smash Diet

The Fat Smash Diet

The Take-Control Diet

Dr. Ian Smith's Guide to Medical Websites

Fiction

The Ancient Nine

The Blackbird Papers

THE Clean20

20 Foods, 20 Days, Total Transformation

Ian K. Smith, M.D.

St. Martin's Griffin ☙ New York

THE CLEAN 20. Copyright © 2018 by Ian K. Smith, M.D. All rights reserved. Printed in the United States of America. For information, address St. Martin's Press, 175 Fifth Avenue, New York, N.Y. 10010.

www.stmartins.com

The Library of Congress has cataloged the hardcover edition as follows:

Names: Smith, Ian K., author.
Title: The clean 20 : 20 foods, 20 days, total transformation / Ian K. Smith, M.D.
Other titles: Clean twenty
Description: First edition. | New York : St. Martin's Press, 2018. | Includes index.
Identifiers: LCCN 2017055140 | ISBN 9781250182074 (hardcover) | ISBN 9781250182067 (ebook)
Subjects: LCSH: Natural foods. | Nutrition. | Food habits. | Exercise.
Classification: LCC TX369 .S63 2018 | DDC 641.3/02—dc23
LC record available at https://lccn.loc.gov/2017055140

ISBN 978-1-250-30978-5 (trade paperback)

Our books may be purchased in bulk for promotional, educational, or business use. Please contact your local bookseller or the Macmillan Corporate and Premium Sales Department at 1-800-221-7945, extension 5442, or by email at MacmillanSpecialMarkets@macmillan.com.

First St. Martin's Griffin Edition: December 2018

10 9 8 7 6 5 4 3 2 1

To Tristè, Dashiell, and Declan—I'd give you the earth, the moon, the sun, and the stars. We keep chasing those rainbows. I love you from the depth of places I never knew existed!

contents

acknowledgments

This is my fifteenth published book and twelve of them have been done at the venerable house of St. Martin's Press. There's a lot of work that goes into publishing and marketing a book that most readers will never know. Yes, the ideas and words start somewhere in the buried neurological tracts of my brain, but by the time you see them, a lot of hands have sculpted the art that finally sits on the shelf or in your digital reader. That means there are a lot of unrecognized heroes who have vastly contributed to the finished works for which they rarely receive their proper due.

So on the occasion of celebrating my fifteenth book, I want to take a moment to honor my partners who have been so generous and instrumental in the arc of my career. They range from publishers and editors to publicists and artists to marketers to the doorman who is nice enough to let me into the Flatiron Building with a welcoming smile and without bureaucratic hassle. Here are their names in no particular order since they all are important to me: Steve Cohen, Elizabeth Beier, Sally Richardson, Jen Enderlin, Matthew Shear, John Karle, John Sargent, Michael Storrings, Louis Krivoshey, Tom Stouras, Lorraine Saullo, John Cusack, Della Cheng, Nicole Williams, Anne Marie Tallberg,

Nancy Trypuc, Brant Janeway, Erica Martirano, Jessica Preeg, Laura Clark, Jeff Dodes, Jeff Capshew, Brian Heller, Jeanette Zwart, Christine Jaeger, Eric C. Meyer, Cheryl Mamaril, Sara Thwaite, Nicola Ferguson, and the St. Martin's super sales team. To all of you and those I might've mistakenly omitted—I extend profound gratitude and the hope that we have another fifteen more creations together. The ride with all its twists and turns has been absolutely AWESOME, and I wouldn't change a thing!

introduction

I was in the gym in the middle of my workout when the idea for *The Clean* 20 came to me. I had spent the previous afternoon with a friend of mine and she was telling me about how sluggish she sometimes felt and how she would love to "get her body back." She had been experimenting with different types of foods to see if she could boost her energy levels, lose weight, and increase her overall sense of feeling good. I'd heard this exact situation described by many people throughout my travels making appearances talking about health and wellness. But the conversation with my friend really struck home for me. On the outside she was pretty, not overweight at all, and seemed to be so much in her groove. But inside there was conflict and doubt and a real struggle that was not allowing her to feel her best or how she knew she could feel.

So there I was in the gym the next morning and she sent me a text. I told her that I had done some research and that I felt comfortable I could customize a meal and exercise plan that could help her. While food can't solve all of our problems, it can solve a lot of them or at least start pointing us in the right direction. The right foods really have medicinal properties. Food can truly affect your physiology—how your body works—and how it interacts with the environment.

The other part of the conversation with my friend centered on exercise. She was exercising, but she was inconsistent, and in my opinion she wasn't doing the optimal exercises to achieve the results she desired. I realized that the foods she was eating or not eating were affecting her energy level and this was in turn affecting her motivation to exercise. It's one of those "which came first, the chicken or the egg?" but it was all making sense to me. She needed to spend less time exercising, but more time exercising efficiently. The hours she spent in the gym didn't matter, but how she spent them could make all the difference in the world.

I modified her exercise plan to go along with her custom-built meal plan. I figured she only needed twenty major foods to fuel her transformation and she needed only twenty minutes of efficient exercise five times a week to synergize with her improved nutritional intake. *The Clean 20* is an expanded version of her plan. There is nothing arbitrary about it, as it is all backed up by science and research. So much of what we put into our body in the form of food or drink is either harmful or counterproductive. We make our bodies work overtime to metabolize and process these foods. We also hamper the body's ability to function at its best. With *The Clean 20*, you are going to change things around and give your body what it needs to operate like the magnificent machine it was built to be. In just twenty days you will have a physical, mental, and spiritual transformation that can last you a lifetime!

Ian K. Smith, M.D.
April 2018

Part I

The Foundation

one

What Is Clean Eating?

Clean eating is a concept and term that has been around for decades but has become fashionable in the last several years as health trends in general have gained popularity from being promoted in reality shows to fitness centers to tiny kitchens across the country. In its simplest form, clean eating is based on the basic premise that eating more natural, less-processed foods is not only good for one's health, but equally important for the environment. Food that crosses our table in a form closest to what it looked like coming out of the ground or off a tree has been considered to be the healthiest and the natural order of humankind's engagement with the environment. Free of chemicals, artificial ingredients, and other potentially toxic additives, clean food represents the best there is to nourish and fuel our bodies.

The clean-eating movement, like any other popular trend (paleo, gluten-free, raw) has not been immune to detractors who claim that it unfairly demonizes certain food groups, takes the concept of avoiding processed foods to the extreme, is too expensive, and is impractical for most people to follow for an extended period of time. It has given birth to many derivative programs that fall under the general category of clean eating but have subtle and sometimes major differences in philosophy and execution strategies. Ask fifteen nutritionists to define clean eating and you are likely to get fifteen different answers. But there is a theme that runs through most of these answers, a common core that gives form to the basic concept of eating foods in their most natural state with as little manipulation as possible.

In *The Clean 20*, I will set forth some basic clean-eating principals that will serve you well and help you make informed decisions when it comes to nourishing the world's most awesome machine—your body. Clean eating is not at all about perfection. It is not about a rigid, dense cadre of rules and penalties that must be strictly adhered to in order to benefit from the tremendous health value of food. Clean eating can benefit all of us and at the same time not be overly expensive, overly restrictive, or inaccessible. Remember that some of a good thing is still better than none of a good thing, and to think harshly of those who do not believe in austere eating principles is a misplaced judgment.

Reducing Processed Foods

Despite what some purists think, not all processed foods are bad for you and some processed foods still can fall under the category of clean foods. The term "processed" is considered to be the equivalent of unhealthy by many, and for good reason. Take grains, for example. In their processing methods, manufacturers will take the whole grain and refine, mill, or process it by taking away part or parts of the three-part grain (bran, endosperm, germ). This could mean losing as many as fifteen or more different nutrients. Once the manufacturers have stripped the grain, they then use a process to add some—but not all—of the nutrients back. This is where the word "enriched," which you may have seen on bread or cracker packaging, comes from. This is why it's better to choose an "unrefined" grain over a "refined" grain and it's important to pay attention to labels such as "100% whole grain" or "100% whole wheat." When it comes to bread, that 100% makes a big difference. Multigrain might seem like the same thing, but it's not: multigrain simply means many grains. This is not a guarantee that grains are whole. You could still be eating many grains that are refined.

HULL:
Inedible outer layer

BRAN:
Outer skin, protects the seed
- B Vitamins
- Fiber
- Trace Minerals

ENDOSPERM:
Middle Layer, provides energy
- B Vitamins
- Carbohydrates
- Protein

GERM:
Nutrient rich core
- Antioxidants
- B Vitamins
- Healthy Fats
- Trace Minerals
- Vitamin E

ANATOMY OF A WHOLE GRAIN

There is no hard and fast rule when it comes to how many ingredients should be in a clean food, but many nutritionists suggest that if a product has more than five or six ingredients, then it's likely not to be very "clean." It's easy to look at the food label and check the ingredients list. If a package does not have a list of ingredients and you aren't certain of what it contains, it's prudent to either confirm the information or approach the product with a fair degree of caution.

Decreasing Added Sugars

Plenty of foods naturally contain sugar. Fruits, for example, should be part of the foundation of any good eating regimen, and many fruits contain lots of natural sugars. (Some have less sugar: apples, avocados, blackberries, grapefruit, peaches, oranges, raspberries, strawberries.) What a lot of people don't know is that many vegetables also naturally contain sugar. Peppers, carrots, parsnips, radishes, squash, potatoes, corn, and peas are just a few examples of sugar-containing vegetables. Demanding all clean foods be free of sugar is nonsensical, as that would mean eliminating fruits and vegetables that are the staples of any healthy diet.

But what does make sense is eliminating foods that have *added* sugars. In the course of processing foods, manufacturers are keen to add sugar to the mix. This makes complete sense from a business perspective, as sugar is highly satisfying to the palate and addictive. If people like the sugar and it will sell, then give them the sugar; health consequences typically take a back seat to the financial concerns. The major food and beverage sources that contain added sugars include candy, cakes, cookies, donuts, pastries, sweet rolls, pies, sodas or soft drinks, energy drinks, sports drinks, and fruit drinks such as fruitades and fruit punch.

A study published in *JAMA Internal Medicine* found that added sugars make up at least 10% of the calories the average American eats in a day. But approximately one in ten people get an enormous 25% of their calories from added sugar. Why does this matter? Because the findings of this study were earthshattering. Over the course of this fifteen-year study, participants who took in 25% or more of their daily calories as sugar were more than twice as likely to die from heart disease compared to those who included less than 10% added sugar in their diets. The study went one step further and concluded that the odds of dying from heart disease rose in tandem with the percentage of sugar in the diet, something that was true regardless of a person's age, sex, physical activity level, or body-mass index (BMI).

It's important when looking at labels to be able to identify these added sugars. The ingredients list is created in a specific way. Ingredients are listed in descending order, which means the closer it is to the front of the list the higher a percentage it is in the food. But you must be careful. Just because you might see sugar listed as the fifth ingredient doesn't mean it is not the ingredient with the highest percentage. Sugars have lots of different names, many of which you are not going to recognize. So, if the ingredients list has corn syrup as number three, dextrose as number five, cane sugar as number six, and malted barley as number eight, then there's a good chance that when you add all of those together, they will actually make sugar the number one ingredient.

Identifying these sugars and sorting through all their confusing names can be very tricky. Here is a good list to use, but note that there are other names manufacturers might be using to sneak that sugar into your food. This list is not comprehensive, but it is a great place to start:

- anhydrous dextrose
- brown sugar
- cane sugar
- carbitol
- confectioners' powdered sugar
- corn syrup
- corn syrup solids
- dextrose
- disaccharide
- evaporated cane sugar
- fructose
- galactose
- glucitol
- glucosamine
- glucose
- hexitol
- high-fructose corn syrup (HFCS)
- honey
- inversol
- invert sugar
- isomalt
- lactose
- malted barley
- maltodextrin
- maltose
- malt syrup
- mannitol
- maple syrup
- molasses
- monosaccharide
- nectars (e.g., peach nectar, pear nectar)
- pancake syrup
- pentose
- polysaccharide
- raisin syrup
- raw sugar
- refiners
- rice malt
- rice sugar
- sorbitol
- sorghum
- Sucanat
- sucanet
- sucrose
- sugar
- white granulated sugar
- xylitol
- zylose

Reducing Unnecessary Additives

"Additive" is a term that encompasses an extremely large number of food ingredients. In its simplest and broadest definition, a food additive is any substance that is added to food. Its more legal definition: "any substance the intended use of which results or may reasonably be expected to result—directly or indirectly—in its becoming a component or otherwise affecting the characteristics of any food." Direct food additives are those that are added to a food for a specific purpose in that food. Xanthan gum is a good example, as it's often used in foods such as bakery fillings, puddings, and salad dressings to add texture and prevent ingredients from separating. Most direct additives are identified on ingredient labels.

Indirect food additives are those that become part of the food in very small amounts due to the process of packaging, storing, or other handling methods. Regardless of how sanitary or expertly manufactured, small amounts of substances that are part of packaging can actually end up in the food. This is why food packaging manufacturers are required to prove to the U.S. Food and Drug Administration (FDA) that all materials that come into contact with the food are safe before they're allowed to be used.

Most food coloring or color additives certainly do not pass muster for a food that is considered to be clean. (There are, however, some natural colorings such as annatto, betanin, cochineal extract, carmine, and chlorophyllin that would meet the clean eating standard.) These coloring additives are dyes, pigments, or substances such as Blue No. 1, Blue No. 2, and Red No. 3 that are capable of imparting color when added or applied to a food, drug, cosmetic, or human body. Without color additives, colas wouldn't be brown and mint ice cream wouldn't be green. Almost all the processed foods we eat contain some color additives. In fact, without color additives we wouldn't recognize the vast majority of the foods we are accustomed to eating.

Food preservatives are natural or man-made chemicals that are added to foods to stop them from spoiling. Preservatives have been used for centuries, most famously salt to preserve fish and meats. Preservatives often have an acidic quality and largely work by preventing the growth of organisms such as molds, yeast, and bacteria. Without preservatives, our food would spoil quickly and be overrun with microorganisms that could cause illness if consumed. There is a surprisingly large number of foods that contain preservatives, everything from soft drinks to cheese, dried fruit to processed meats. While some preservatives are necessary to sustain food, there is plenty of preservatives, such as monosodium glutamate (MSG), propyl gallate, potassium bromate, and many more, that could have harmful health consequences.

Try to limit the amount of preservatives in your food; start by reading the nutrition labels carefully. Cleaner foods don't have these additives, so it's true that in general they might spoil faster than processed foods. But this is not a reason to choose the additive-rich foods. Making smart choices at the right time of the season means you will still be able to purchase clean products that will last at least through most of the week, thus reducing the need for you to go grocery shopping multiple times in a single week.

Following is a list of commonly used preservatives that you should try to avoid. By no means is this a comprehensive list, but it is a good place to start:

- butylated hydroxyanisole (BHA)
- butylated hydroxytoluene (BHT)
- potassium benzoate
- propyl gallate
- sodium benzoate
- sodium nitrate
- tertiary butylhydroquinone (TBHQ)

The FDA is responsible for regulating food coloring as well as other additives, but the FDA is not perfect and has its limitations with regard to budget and other resources. Its major goal is to make sure that these additives are generally regarded as safe. However, expecting a single governmental agency to be able to know everything there is to know about these ingredients and their long-term health implications is unrealistic. In fact, these safety clearances are quite dynamic, as new information and studies may emerge that show that something previously listed as safe is no longer as safe as once thought. Ingredients are constantly coming on and off the list of accepted additives or finding themselves under additional review. So, while the FDA is a good place to start when trying to ascertain the safety of additives, finding other resources is necessary for a more exhaustive analysis.

Clean eating is all about knowing what you're putting in your body and the impact foods and beverages can have on not just your health, but your mind and overall functioning. It comes down to making smarter, strategic choices, being aware not only of the ingredients you're consuming but how these ingredients are harvested, processed, and packaged. The overall goal is to consume minimally processed foods that are nutritionally dense (relatively rich in nutrients for a lower number of calories), affordable, tasty, and good for the environment. Clean eating can be not only a blueprint for the next twenty days, but one you can follow for the rest of your life.

two

- - - - - - - - - - - - - - - - - - - -

The Clean 20 Foods

Over the next twenty days you are going to eat foods that are clean and full of nature's best health-promoting nutrients. You will only need twenty foods to complete the plan, but that does not mean that you are restricted to those twenty. If you want to have more, by all means, go ahead and do so, but with one caveat: any foods that you choose that are not on the original Clean 20 list must fit the guidelines of the program. The Clean 20 list that I created (see page 16) does not have to be your list. For some of the items there are other options you can choose to eat. Those options are in parentheses and called "Basket Buddies." There is also a secondary list. This list is for the different types of herbs and spices and other "non-major food groups" you might want to use during these twenty days. This list is not meant to be comprehensive, so if you don't see a spice or herb that you want to use, don't feel like it is forbidden. If it's natural and not processed with artificial ingredients, feel free to go ahead and eat it. You will be consuming a significant amount of phytonutrients (plant nutrients) over the next twenty days that include vitamins and minerals. These powerful health boosters are critical to life and your total transformation.

CLEAN 20 Minerals

Calcium	Makes bones and teeth; helps with muscle contraction/relaxation, nerve function, blood clotting, and blood pressure maintenance.
Chromium	Helps insulin move glucose from the blood into the cells.
Copper	Aids digestion and absorption; lubricates joints and organs; regulates body temperature.
Iodine	Component of thyroid hormone—regulates growth, development, and metabolism.
Iron	Part of hemoglobin molecule; carries oxygen in the blood.
Magnesium	Helps with mineralization of bones and teeth, muscle contraction, nerve conduction, enzyme function.
Phosphorus	Helps maintain bones and teeth; important in our DNA and cell membranes; helps body get energy from food.
Selenium	Antioxidant that works with vitamin E and fights damaging particles in the body called free radicals.
Sodium	Controls fluid balance; assists nerve impulse transmission and muscle contractions.
Zinc	Helps many enzymes function properly; part of insulin molecule; helps DNA repair as well as immune function, wound healing, and taste perception.

CLEAN 20 Vitamins

Vitamin A (Retinol)	Improves eyesight; helps with bone growth and reproduction; regulates immune system; helps with appetite and taste.
Vitamin B1 (Thiamine)	Part of enzyme needed for energy metabolism; important for nerve, muscle, and heart function as well as digestion.

Vitamin B2 (Riboflavin)	Important for normal vision and skin health as well as nails and eyesight; helps with breakdown of fat and carbohydrates.
Vitamin B3 (Niacin)	Important for digestive system, nervous system, and skin health.
Vitamin B5 (Pantothenic Acid)	Plays a role in the breakdown of fats and carbohydrates for energy; important for manufacture of red blood cells as well as sex and stress-related hormones produced in adrenal glands.
Vitamin B6 (Pyridoxine)	Needed for protein metabolism; helps make red blood cells and prevent nerve and skin conditions.
Vitamin B9 (Folic Acid)	Part of an enzyme needed for making DNA and new cells, particularly red blood cells; essential in first three months of pregnancy to prevent spina bifida, cleft palate, and cleft lip.
Vitamin B12 (Cobalamin)	Needed for making new cells; important to nerve function.
Vitamin C (Ascorbic Acid)	Antioxidant that fights toxins; part of an enzyme needed for protein metabolism; helps with iron absorption; important for immune system health.
Vitamin D	Needed for proper absorption of calcium; important for strong bones and teeth.
Vitamin E (Tocopherol)	Antioxidant that fights toxins; protects cell wall from damage; supports immune function and DNA repair.
Vitamin K	Need for the blood to clot properly.

Take your time as you form your initial Clean 20 list. You might even look in the back of the book in the recipes section and mark some you definitely want to try, then look at the ingredients and add them to your list if they aren't already on it. This list is your blueprint, so make sure you create it thoughtfully and realistically. This is your list, so there are items that you might include on your main list that I don't. For example, you might want apples and pears but not berries. Not a problem, just look at the "Basket Buddies" and choose whatever and how many you want from that group.

The Clean 20 Food List

Avocados

Berries (*Basket Buddies: apples, pears, mangos, bananas, watermelon, honeydew melon, cantaloupe, oranges*)

Cheese

Chicken

Chickpeas (*Basket Buddies: black beans, red beans, cannellini beans, pinto beans, lima beans, black-eyed peas, peas, corn*)

Eggs

Kale (*Basket Buddies: arugula, bok choy, brussels sprouts, cabbage, cauliflower, collard greens, spinach, swiss chard, watercress*)

Lemons (*Basket Buddies: limes, grapefruit*)

Lentils

Nuts (*Basket Buddies: sunflower seeds, pumpkin seeds, chia seeds, hemp seeds, flax seeds*)

Oatmeal (*Basket Buddies: grits*)

Seafood (*Basket Buddies: cod, crab, halibut, lobster, oysters, salmon, sea bass, shrimp, tuna*)

Squash (*Basket Buddies: broccoli, carrots, cucumbers, eggplant, parsnips, zucchini*)

Sweet potatoes (*Basket Buddies: corn*)

Tomatoes

Turkey

Quinoa

100% whole-grain or whole-wheat bread

Whole-wheat pasta

Yogurt

Spices, Herbs, and Others

Balsamic vinegar (*Basket Buddies: apple cider vinegar, rice vinegar, white wine vinegar*)

Basil

Cumin

Extra-virgin olive oil (*Basket Buddies: avocado oil, grapeseed oil, sesame oil*)

Garlic

Ginger

Granola (organic, no preservatives or artificial ingredients, no sugar added)

Milk (organic, unsweetened fat-free or low-fat or 1%, 2%, almond, coconut)

Oregano

Organic honey

Organic mayonnaise

Organic peanut butter (*Basket Buddies: almond nut butter, cashew nut butter, sunflower seed butter*)

Organic soy sauce

Paprika

Parsley

Pepper

Rosemary

Saffron

Sage

Salt

Thyme

Turmeric

1 AVOCADO

The avocado is the fattiest fruit you will find (almost 75%), out-pacing the olive, which also contains a significant amount of healthy fat. While "fat" is often regarded as a bad word, not so when it comes to the avocado. Most of the fat buried in its creamy flesh is monounsaturated—the good kind that has heart-protective properties because it helps lower the LDL ("bad") cholesterol levels. While this fat is very healthy for you, calorie-conscious consumers must beware, because an avocado packs as many as 120 to 150 calories in just half a cup.

Avocados are stuffed with many nutrients, including vitamins B5, folate, K, B6, E, and C. They're also a good source of fiber, copper, potassium, and manganese. Buried in its flesh, you'll find other phytonutrients such as carotenoids, flavonoids, and phy-tosterols that have antioxidant and anti-inflammatory proper-ties. If you're carb conscious, don't worry about the numbers. While an avocado contains 9 grams of carbs per every 3.5 ounce serving, 7 of those carbs are fiber, so in actuality there are only 2 "net" grams of carbs. The other good news—avocados don't contain any cholesterol or sodium.

There are hundreds of avocado varieties—Bacon, Cocktail, Fuerte, Gwen, Lula, Pinterton, Reed, Zutano, and many more—but the most common is Hass, which originated in California and is also grown in Florida. This is the most popular avocado variety grown around the world and is often called the "year-round avocado" because it can be grown in some places the entire calendar year or imported from other countries. These avocados are oval-shaped, with a distinctive bumpy skin that turns from green to purplish black when ripe. Their seed—the hard core—is small- to medium-sized and the fruit typically weighs between 5 and 12 ounces.

Avocados can be enjoyed in a variety of preparations. Slice them and add them to salad, mash them to make guacamole, chunk and throw them into a smoothie, or enjoy them spread thickly on toast. Their rich taste and creamy texture are undeniable and they can add powerful flavor to any dish. It's also important to note that avocados do not ripen on the tree; rather, they soften after they've been harvested. Contrary to popular belief, the microwave is not an effective method of speeding up the ripening process. This is why avocados should be purchased at least a couple of days before you are actually going to use them.

AVOCADO BENEFITS

- Full of monounsaturated fats.
- Rich source of potassium (more than bananas).
- Loaded with fiber.
- Increases body absorption of vitamins A, D, E, and K and antioxidants, thus increasing nutrient value of other plant foods.
- Helps maintain eye health (via lutein and zeaxanthin).
- Could assist weight loss because it keeps you full longer.

2 BERRIES (BLUEBERRIES, RASPBERRIES, AND STRAWBERRIES)

Berries are some of the world's most powerful superfoods. They are nutritional dynamite, bursting with a tremendous amount of nutrition that delivers so many health benefits for few calories. While there are differences among the various berries, they share similar nutritional profiles and can be easily found at most grocery stores or farmers' markets.

Berries are considered one of the best superfoods because they are low in calories and outrageously nutritious. They contain a very high level of antioxidants that directly impact health. Antioxidants are compounds that neutralize potentially dangerous unstable molecules in your body called "free radicals" that can damage your cells when too many are present. In addition to protecting your cells, these abundant compounds may help reduce the risk of disease.

When people think of vitamin C, they typically think of oranges and orange juice, but they are underestimating the punch of berries. Strawberries, in particular, are loaded with vitamin C. One cup contains 150% of the recommended daily intake or daily value (DV), which is slightly higher than oranges, and it delivers that vitamin C in fewer calories. Vitamin C is the only major difference in the nutritional profile of the berry types, as they are very similar with regards to their overall vitamin and mineral offerings. Strawberries lead the way, while blueberries and cranberries trail far behind at 16% DV and 22% DV, respectively.

Berries also rank high among superfoods because, along with all of the vitamins (A, B-complex, C, K) and other minerals (iron, selenium, manganese, copper, magnesium, potassium, and zinc), they contain a relatively significant amount of fiber, which can slow the movement of food through the digestive tract, thus reducing hunger and increasing feelings of fullness. Here are the fiber counts per 1 cup of berries: blackberries: 8 grams; raspberries: 8 grams; blueberries: 4 grams; strawberries: 3 grams.

When it comes to choosing berries, you simply can't go wrong. Widely available, convenient to transport, and easy to store, berries also offer great flexibility. Eat them by themselves as a snack, or throw them into smoothies, muffins, yogurt, salads, soups, and sauces.

BERRIES BENEFITS

- Help prevent heart disease.
- Helpful with weight loss due to fiber and high liquid content.
- Low in calories.
- Full of anthocyanidins, compounds that could help slow mental decline of aging.
- Cranberries and blueberries can help fight urinary tract infections.
- Could lower chances of developing Parkinson's by 25%.
- Could reduce cancer risk due to the high content of flavonoids.

SHOPPING/HANDLING

- Cheaper and more available when in season (strawberry season is May to August; blackberry, raspberry, and blueberry is June to September).
- You can purchase fresh berries and usually freeze them safely for up to a year (if using them for smoothies, freeze in a bag, but if using them to eat individually, freeze in one layer on a baking sheet).
- The fruit should be plump but firm with intense color and no mold or disfigurement.
- Rinse right before use, not too far in advance.
- Nutritional benefits are stronger when eaten whole rather than in another food.

3 CHEESE

Such a daunting food category, it's almost difficult to know where to start in extolling its virtues. Taste is probably as good a place as any to explain why this food has been extremely popular and in demand around the world for thousands of years. Regardless of the type of cheese—and there are hundreds of them—it all starts with the one ingredient: milk. Cheese makers will unanimously tell you that all quality cheese begins with quality milk. And it takes a lot of milk—approximately 10 pounds to make 1 pound of cheese!

Beyond its great taste and vast assortment to choose from, cheese's nutritional profile stands tall. While different varieties will have different nutritional qualities, there are several universal elements that make it a smart choice on our program. Protein tops the list. For example, one thick slice of cheddar cheese (28 grams) contains almost 7 grams of protein. This is approximately what you would expect to get from an entire glass of milk. Most of these proteins belong to a family of milk proteins called casein. They are rich in essential amino acids, highly digestible (for most people), and of excellent quality.

Cheese also contains a wide array of vitamins and minerals. Chief among minerals is calcium, a mineral that many of us don't consume enough of on a daily basis. To give you better context, the recommended daily allowance (RDA) of calcium according to the National Institutes of Health (NIH) is as follows:

Age	Male	Female	Pregnant	Lactating
0–6 months*	200 mg	200 mg		
7–12 months*	260 mg	260 mg		
1–3 years	700 mg	700 mg		
4–8 years	1,000 mg	1,000 mg		
9–13 years	1,300 mg	1,300 mg		
14–18 years	1,300 mg	1,300 mg	1,300 mg	1,300 mg
19–50 years	1,000 mg	1,000 mg	1,000 mg	1,000 mg
51–70 years	1,000 mg	1,200 mg		
71+ years	1,200 mg	1,200 mg		

* Adequate intake (AI)

One ounce of cheddar cheese supplies you with as much as 204 milligrams, mozzarella has 222 milligrams per ounce, and Swiss contains 224 milligrams. Most people are aware that calcium is important for bone and tooth health, but what many don't know is that it's critical for many other physiologic processes in the body, including narrowing and widening blood vessels, nerve transmission, muscle function, and chemical signaling between the billions of cells in our body. Simply put, calcium is the most abundant mineral in our body and we need lots of it to stay healthy.

Cheese also is a rich source of vitamin A, vitamin B12, phosphorous, and zinc. Depending on the variety of cheese and how it was prepared, the amount of these specific nutrients will vary, but generally you can expect to find this cluster of vitamins and minerals present to some degree.

The taste of cheese is an individual preference, so it's pointless to try to parse out which cheese tastes better than others. But it *does* make sense to talk about some of the healthiest cheeses on the planet.

Cottage cheese: High in protein, low in fat, and flexible in its use. You only consume 20 calories for a 1-ounce serving, but you get 3 grams of protein and a high amount of calcium along with it.

Feta: A key ingredient in Greek cuisine, it's lower in fat and calories than most cheese and has 4 grams of protein in only a 1-ounce serving. Typically made from sheep's milk or a combination of sheep's and goat's milk, its flavor is so strong you can typically get away with less, which means consuming fewer calories.

Mozzarella: Only 70 calories per ounce, it offers 5 grams of protein and only 5 grams of fat.

Parmesan: Relatively low in calories with 110 per 1-ounce serving, it has a big kick of flavor, which means you don't need much to get the job done. A whopping 10 grams of protein come along for the ride, and it also contains umami, a "fifth" taste in food (the other four are bitter, salty, sweet, and sour) that comes from glutamate and makes foods taste better and potentially improves digestion and gut health. Foods with natural umami include carrots, chicken, mushrooms, shellfish, soy, tomatoes, and tuna.

Ricotta: Half a cup contains 14 grams of protein and 25% of your daily calcium intake recommendation. It also stands out for being low in sodium while high in vitamin A, B vitamins, phosphorous, and zinc.

CHEESE BENEFITS

- Helps maintain strong teeth via high calcium content.
- Helps form strong bones via calcium and vitamin B.
- Helps fight osteoporosis (bone thinning).
- High in phosphorus, which is important for bone health.
- Source of the all-important vitamin D.

SHOPPING/HANDLING

- Unlike some foods, often quality and price are in line with each other in the cheese world.
- Read the label for cues to help you distinguish between hard, soft, creamy, aged, robust.
- Choose a cheese based on use: for example, Swiss, American, and cheddar are better for melting; Parmesan is better for grating.
- Always wrap it well when storing and use fresh wrapping.
- Avoid freezing cheese or dishes with cheese in them, as you risk losing texture and flavor profile.

4 CHICKEN

Likely to have been domesticated first for cockfights rather than food, the chicken is the most abundant species of bird in the world, topping the ranks at over 25 billion. The terminology can get a bit confusing, but it's pretty straightforward. Baby chickens are called chicks. Female chickens are called pullets, but when they're old enough to lay eggs they become hens. Male chickens are called either cocks, cockerels, or roosters depending on the country they're living in.

Chicken is a great alternative to beef for those looking to consume protein, but at the same time reduce their consumption of red meat. Just a 3.5-ounce serving of skinless, boneless chicken breast yields a whopping 31 grams of protein (beef has 32 to 33 grams) at a cost of only 165 calories. It is an impressively lean meat with only 2 grams of fat, most of it falling into the healthy unsaturated category.

Protein might be chicken's claim to health fame, but there's more nutrition packed in that tender meat. Chicken is an excellent source of vitamin B3 and a very good source of selenium, phosphorus, choline, vitamin B5, and vitamin B6.

Chicken is arguably the most versatile of meats in how it can be prepared, served, and spiced. Roasting and frying (the unhealthiest cooking method and not to be done on the Clean 20 plan) are common preparations in the United States, while in Spain combining it with shellfish and rice creates the popular paella dish. Italians have perfected its preparation by sautéing it with mushrooms, tomatoes, and wine in their classic cacciatore.

Shopping for the healthiest chicken seems to have gotten more complicated in the last ten years or so. There are so many different types of labeling that aren't defined on the packaging. Here are some common terms that you will encounter, but when in doubt, if there is a knowledgeable butcher present, ask him or her to explain how the chicken was raised.

Pasture/pasture raised: This is one of the best labels to look for. It suggests that the chicken lived on a pasture with constant access to edible vegetation. These chickens also get a portion of their food from grass, seeds, and bugs from the natural environment.

Naturally raised: These chickens never receive antibiotics, hormones, or feed containing animal by-products.

Free-range: Throughout their life cycle, these chickens have access to outdoors for at least part of the day. This is a good thing. But the caveat is that this doesn't guarantee that the chickens actually take advantage of this opportunity and go outside. All chickens that are labeled "organic" must also be "free-range," but not all "free-range" chickens are "organic."

Organic: The use of this term is highly regulated by the USDA. It can only be used when no pesticides, chemical fertilizers, or genetically modified organisms (GMOs; foods engineered in a laboratory) are used in the poultry feed, and no antibiotics are used at any stage of the chicken's development or production. The caveat here is that while many are attracted to the word "organic" because it's typically attached to superior quality, it still doesn't mean that it is necessarily the best quality of meat, as there are other factors to consider, such as where the animal was raised and conditions in which it was kept. But the stamp of organic is a sign that the meat is cleanest and free from the unwanted additives that come with processing.

Cage-free: The birds are allowed to freely roam a building, room, or enclosed area. These conditions are often cramped, and the chickens may or may not have outdoor access.

No antibiotics: This certifies that the animal never received antibiotic medications that are commonly used to prevent disease and/or enhance growth.

CHICKEN BENEFITS

- Contains all the B vitamins as well as copper, iron, magnesium, phosphorous, and zinc.
- Loaded with protein.
- Can help with weight-loss efforts.
- Helpful in controlling blood pressure (grilled, baked, or roasted, *not* fried).
- Lowers risk of elevated cholesterol and related heart disease.
- Inexpensive and widely available.
- When skinless, much lower in fat compared to meats with comparable protein.

SHOPPING/HANDLING

- Check for USDA Grade A rating on packaging.
- Choose chicken with creamy white to deep yellow skin.
- Avoid chicken with gray or pasty-looking meat.
- Stay away from chicken with a strong, unpleasant odor.
- Choose organic, pasture-raised, or naturally raised if available.
- Store immediately in coldest part of the refrigerator.
- Keep chicken in its original store wrapping.
- Wash all utensils or objects that come in contact with raw chicken before using.
- Raw chicken will keep in home refrigerator for 2 to 3 days.
- Cooked chicken will keep for 3 to 4 days.

No hormones: It's great that the animal has not been exposed to hormones, but this is almost a useless label, because in 1959 the use of growth hormones in poultry was banned by the U.S. government.

5 CHICKPEAS (GARBANZO BEANS)

This irregular-shaped bean originated in the Middle East around 3000 B.C. and is a staple in Middle Eastern cuisine. Carried to lands all over the world, this legume is enjoyed for its nutty flavor, buttery texture, and versatility. Grown best during winter in tropical and/or subtropical climates over a period of approximately three months, this inexpensive vegetable packs a huge nutritional punch with minimal calories.

There are two primary varieties—Kabuli and Desi, names that have their roots in India. The Kabuli are larger (twice the size of Desi), whitish beige, uniform, and rounded in shape. The Kabuli-type chickpeas are the most common here in the United States, though not so in the rest of the world. Desi chickpeas are not only smaller, but darker in color, ranging from a light tan to black. They are more irregular in shape and have a thicker seed coat.

What many people don't know is that the delicious hummus that you might enjoy as pita, cucumber, or carrot dip is actually made from mashed chickpeas. This is an extremely versatile vegetable that can be added to a variety of dishes, including salads, soups, or stir-fries. Many vegetarians looking for a good source of nonanimal protein often turn to chickpeas.

Chickpeas are also favored for their high fiber content, something that's important to help stabilize blood sugar levels, minimize cholesterol absorption, and enhance the functionality of your digestive system. Just consuming one cup can provide half of your entire daily recommended intake. Beyond fiber there's a significant amount of protein, vitamin B6 (folate), zinc, and

CHICKPEAS BENEFITS

- Increases feeling of fullness.
- Boosts digestion.
- Great source of fiber.
- Great source of protein.
- Great source of antioxidants.
- Reduces unhealthy cholesterol.
- High in vitamin B6 (folate).

- Source of vitamin C.
- Source of zinc.
- Source of magnesium.
- Source of manganese.
- Source of iron.
- Source of potassium.
- Source of phosphorous.

SHOPPING/HANDLING

- If buying from a bulk bin, make sure bin is covered.
- If packaged, make sure there's no moisture or insect damage.
- Make sure the bean seeds are not cracked, but are whole.
- Store dried beans in airtight container in cool, dry, dark place for up to 1 year.
- Cooked beans can last for about 3 days in the refrigerator.
- If using canned beans, check the sodium levels to make sure they are not high (140 milligrams or less per serving).
- If using dried beans, make sure you soak and drain them before cooking.

antioxidants, as well as other vitamins and minerals that are essential for good health.

More good news is how easy it is to cook and use this nutritional legume. You can purchase them in a can or in their raw dried form. Boiling or roasting them and adding some spices is about all it takes to get the most out of this versatile legume. They can be cooked with almost anything, given their ability to absorb the flavors of other foods. You can add them to a salad concoction, make them a part of your soup, mash them up into a tasty hummus that can be spread on pita, or roast them with spices. This is one vegetable that is really good and extremely convenient in its canned form, as it doesn't have to be peeled or prepared in any major way. You will not be disappointed with all that chickpeas offer, and incorporating them into your meal plans will be effortless.

6 EGGS

Eggs are one of the most nutritious foods on the planet, especially when you consider their cost relative to other nutrient-dense foods. They contain some of almost every nutrient we need for good health. Among their many nutrients you'll find vitamins A, B2, B5, B6, B9 (folate), D, E, and K as well as calcium, phosphorus, selenium, and zinc. However, they have not been free from controversy, largely because of the amount of cholesterol they contain. A large egg contains approximately 186 milligrams of cholesterol while a small egg contains 141 milligrams. To put this in context, the American Heart Association recommends healthy adults consume no more than 300 milligrams per day. Excess cholesterol has been implicated in heart disease, so it has been the counsel of most medical professionals and health advocates to monitor cholesterol intake and blood levels.

While health professionals and researchers continue to sift through the conflicting information about eggs and their cholesterol, there are some issues where a general consensus has been reached. Cholesterol is not all bad for the body, and in fact it is needed in certain quantities. Not only do we consume cholesterol in our foods, but it's also naturally made by the liver. For most people, consuming eggs doesn't increase total cholesterol levels, because the liver will decrease its natural production of cholesterol to counteract the increase in cholesterol that comes from eating. Research has also shown that while eggs can increase cholesterol levels, they predominantly increase the good cholesterol, otherwise known as HDL. Higher levels of HDL can help the body get rid of the unhealthy LDL cholesterol (bad cholesterol) and can contribute to reducing a person's risk for heart disease and stroke.

Differentiating the quality of eggs can be extremely challenging. Here is a simple guideline to help.

Color: The color of an egg's shell has nothing to do with its nutritional benefits. Color is based on the hen's breed and genetics. Some hens even lay blue and green eggs, but they don't show up at the store, because many consumers would be unlikely to buy them!

Animal welfare approved: This has one of the most rigorous standards for farm animal welfare and environmental sustainability currently in use by the U.S. farm program. This labeling requires audited, high-welfare slaughter practices and pasture access for all animals. Hens must be cage-free with continual access to outdoor perching and ability to engage in natural behaviors, such as nesting, spreading wings, dust bathing, and so on. Beak cutting is prohibited.

Cage-free: There are currently no national standards for cage-free egg production in the United States, but the term usually means the hens are not in cages (though still indoors). Cage-free is considered more humane than the crowded cages that house the majority of egg-laying hens in the United States—because cage-free hens may have more room to walk and spread their wings, for example—but the birds may still be subject to other questionable practices, such as beak cutting.

Certified humane: These eggs are from hens that are not caged and must have enough space to engage in natural behaviors—but they may be indoors all the time. And beak cutting is still allowed. There is third-party auditing for compliance.

Certified organic: These are eggs that come from hens that have been fed certified organically grown vegetarian feed. The feed must not contain any pesticides, hormones, antibiotics, or pesticides. The hens are not caged and must have access to outdoors—however, the length of time outdoors and the quality of the space is not defined. Moreover, forced molting (artificially provoking a flock to molt or lose their feathers simultaneously) and beak cutting (to prevent animals from harming one another) are still permitted. If you choose to buy organic, look for the USDA Organic seal. Keep in mind, though, that organic eggs aren't necessarily safer from bacteria than other eggs; it depends on the sanitation conditions of that farm and other factors. Nor are they more nutritious than conventionally produced ones.

Free-range or free-roaming: Hens are not caged and must have access to the outdoors. But just because they have access to the outdoors doesn't necessarily mean that they do go outside. There are no requirements for the amount of time they spend outside or the amount of space provided.

There's often debate about whether to wash eggs. Don't. It actually increases the risk of contamination because water can enter through the porous shell. When laid, eggs have a natural waxy bloom for protection, and washing removes this. Commercially produced eggs are washed and sanitized, then producers apply a thin coating of wax to the shells to protect their porous surface from absorbing bacteria or odors.

EGGS BENEFITS

- Great source of protein.
- Egg whites are rich sources of vitamins B6, B12, and D, as well as copper, iron, selenium, and zinc.
- Raise HDL ("good") cholesterol.
- Contain choline, which is important for building cell membranes and producing signaling molecules in the brain.
- Contain lutein and zeaxanthin—antioxidants that help eye health.

SHOPPING/HANDLING

- The color of the egg—brown or white—doesn't matter; they are nutritionally identical.
- Always check the sell-by date on the carton: eggs are typically good for 4 to 6 weeks after this date if they are properly refrigerated.
- Always strive to reduce contamination, so open the carton to make sure none of the eggs are cracked; if one cracks on the trip from the store to your home, throw it away.
- Eggs produced more humanely tend to be more expensive; if you can afford to buy them and desire to do so, you will be a more conscientious consumer.
- Buy eggs graded "large" for use in recipes—that's the standard size used when recipes are tested.
- Temperature is critical to egg safety: store eggs in the coldest part of the refrigerator in their original carton, not in those little egg cups that some refrigerators have in the door.

7 KALE *(BASKET BUDDIES: ARUGULA, BOK CHOY, BRUSSELS SPROUTS, CABBAGE, CAULIFLOWER, COLLARD GREENS, SPINACH, SWISS CHARD, WATERCRESS)*

Kale is a superfood and has been on top of the clean eating charts for some time now. While its popularity has surged within the last decade, the truth is that this dark, leafy green goes all the way back to Roman times. Kale is part of the cabbage or cruciferous family, which includes bok choy, broccoli, brussels sprouts, collards, cauliflower, and garden cress. Unlike many other vegetables, kale actually thrives during the cooler seasons of the year, which can sometimes be reflected in its flavor. Easy to grow, hardy, and inexpensive, kale serves up good nutrition with a broad taste from bitter or even pepper-like to bland or slightly sweet.

Kale has been heralded by health experts for reasons more important than its being just another foodie trend. It contains a long list of vitamins, minerals, and other nutrients. At the top of this list are: forty-five different antioxidant polyphenols (protect against aging and cellular damage), carotenoids, vitamin K, vitamin A, vitamin C, manganese, copper, vitamin B6, fiber, calcium, potassium, iron, vitamin E, vitamin B2, magnesium, vitamin B1, and protein. All of this comes with a very inexpensive price tag—only 33 calories in a cup of chopped kale leaves.

There are several types of kale that have different appearances and different flavors. You won't find all types of kale in your local grocery store, but here are four you're most likely to find. While they may look and taste different, for the most part their nutritional value remains quite similar.

Curly kale: Also called common kale, it's the type you will most often find in grocery stores. Its color ranges from pale to deep green with a slightly bluish hue. It's known for its pungent, almost peppery flavor.

Lacinato-type kale: This type is also known as Dinosaur, Dino, or Tuscan kale with its narrow, wrinkled dark green leaves attached to a hard stem and a stronger flavor.

Premier kale: This variety is easily recognizable with its dark green, smooth flat leaves with scalloped edges; it's full of flavor.

Redbor kale: Visually pleasing with its ruffled leaves ranging in color from deep red to purple, sometimes with

KALE BENEFITS

- Cancer prevention.
- Anti-inflammatory effects.
- Antioxidant properties.
- Reduces cholesterol levels.

SHOPPING/HANDLING

- Try to buy organic to avoid pesticide residue.
- Leaves should not be yellowed or brown.
- If eating raw, choose smaller-leaved kale for tenderness and mild flavor.
- Choose moist, crisp, unwilted leaves without tiny holes.
- Remove the thick center stem to avoid toughness while eating.
- Wrap unwashed kale in damp paper towels, then seal in plastic bag and refrigerate.
- Unwashed kale can be stored in the refrigerator for 5 to 7 days.
- Can be frozen, but blanch first if you want it to keep longer than 6 weeks.

shades of green. This is edible like other kale, but also used ornamentally in gardens and as a garnish.

Kale can be eaten raw like any salad green, stuffed into a blender and made part of a smoothie, lightly cooked in different entrées, and added to soups. Kale can easily be prepared by sautéing it with garlic in extra-virgin olive oil along with other spices such as red pepper flakes, ginger, salt, and pepper. Kale is extremely easy to work with and there are thousands of recipes you can find online or even make up yourself to enjoy this nutritious powerhouse.

8 LEMONS

Lemons are one of the most versatile fruits in the citrus family. Affordable and available around the world, lemons are full of nutrients that can help prevent and fight diseases. Vitamins A, C, B6, E, folate, riboflavin as well as copper, calcium, iron, and magnesium, are just some of the many phytonutrients that make lemons a powerhouse. In fact, while we have historically touted the high levels of vitamin C found in oranges, lemons come in a close second. Oranges contain 50 milligrams of vitamin C per 100 grams of flesh, while lemons contain 40 milligrams. Lemons and their bitter juice have been credited for everything from reducing fever and treating cold symptoms to helping prevent the formation of kidney stones.

Lemon water is a great way to get the nutritional benefits of lemon juice while at the same time hydrating and avoiding calories and carbohydrates. Mixing the juice of half a lemon with a cup of water only means adding 7 calories and 2 grams of carbohydrates, but a full 10 milligrams of vitamin C. Lemon water is great for quenching your thirst and soothing your throat, and has also been shown to suppress appetite.

For those looking for a boost in removing toxins and speeding up important enzymatic reactions in the body, lemons are an answer. Lemon water is believed to play a role in enhancing the enzyme functions in the liver, which increases the rate at which the body eliminates toxins. Lemons are also a slight diuretic, which means they make you urinate: this can be another way to flush unhealthy elements out of your body.

LEMON BENEFITS

- Contains flavonoids, which contain antioxidant, cancer-fighting properties.
- Can help prevent diabetes, constipation, indigestion, high blood pressure, and kidney stones.
- Can treat fever, cold, or flu.
- Has antiseptic and blood-clotting properties.
- Can soothe and relieve respiratory problems.

SHOPPING/HANDLING

- For juicy lemons, choose those that give a little when squeezed and have thinner skin.
- Select lemons that are heavy for their size and have smooth skin that's thin and firm.
- Avoid lemons that have a dull color or are darker yellow, or with skin that is hardened or shriveled.
- Store lemons at room temperature for up to 1 week, or in the refrigerator 2–3 weeks.
- Freeze extra lemons whole to make them juicier.

9 LENTILS *(BASKET BUDDIES: BLACK BEANS, GREEN BEANS, KIDNEY BEANS, WHITE BEANS, SOYBEANS)*

If you're looking for a nutritional powerhouse, you need look no further than the versatile lentil. It belongs to a family of plants called legumes that include beans (soy, kidney, garbanzo/chickpeas, white/cannellini, snap, black, fava, and so on), peanuts, and peas. "Legume" simply refers to plants that grow seeds in a pod. With their nutty flavor and versatility, lentils are tasty, convenient, and great for your health.

Lentils are chock full of nutrition. Since eight to nine thousand years ago in the Middle East, lentils have been an essential foodstuff and traditionally consumed with barley and wheat. The traditional Indian dish dal uses lentils as its main ingredient and is a mainstay particularly for vegetarians. Lentils are full of protein and can help improve heart health, digestion, and diabetes, and prevent atherosclerosis (hardening of the arteries). Lentils also have fiber and many vitamins, particularly the vitamin B-complex such as folate or folic acid, and they are loaded with iron that's important for hemoglobin production in our blood.

Lentils come in many varieties throughout the world. The most common include brown, yellow, green, red, and black. They differ not only in their color, but in their taste, size, and ease of use. Different recipes may call for different types of lentils and these more common varieties are typically easy to find in most grocery stores. Not only are lentils inexpensive, but they are relatively quick and easy to prepare. Whether you want to make soup, salad, or a wrap, you can purchase them precooked in a can or dry in a bag and prepare them as the recipe instructs. Typically, lentils only require 20 to 30 minutes of boiling time, but these times can be adjusted based on how you plan to use them. Contrary to what many think, lentils don't need to be soaked; be careful of overcooking them, as this can make them mushy.

While many canned vegetables tend to lose a significant amount of their nutritional value, there is little loss when comparing canned versus dried lentils. As with any canned vegetables, make sure you purchase a low-sodium preparation. For the purposes of this plan these should also be organic with nothing artificial and no added sugar.

LENTILS BENEFITS

- Good source of nonanimal protein.
- Stabilize blood sugars.
- Reduce cholesterol.
- Loaded with fiber.
- Good source of vitamins B1, 5, 6, and 9.
- Good source of copper, phosphorous, manganese, iron, zinc, potassium.

SHOPPING TIPS

- If purchasing in a can, choose low sodium.
- Purchase in bags or from bulk bins.
- For more selection, try ethnic markets or sections of the grocery store.
- Store dry lentils in airtight containers away from heat and moisture.

10 NUTS AND SEEDS *(OPTIONS: ALMOND, CASHEW, PECANS, PINE, PISTACHIO, PUMPKIN SEEDS, SUNFLOWER SEEDS, WALNUTS)*

Nuts aren't just a tasty and convenient snack; they are full of raw nutrition with a lot of health offerings. For example, take the Global Burden of Disease Study, which is the most comprehensive and systematic analysis of the causes of death ever undertaken. This study combined the efforts of nearly five hundred researchers from more than three hundred institutions, spread across fifty countries. Among other things, the study looked at which foods could save lives if added to the diet. Researchers calculated that eating more nuts could potentially save 2.5 million lives. It also calculated that not eating enough nuts and seeds was the third leading dietary risk factor for death and disability in the world.

There are more than fifty varieties of nuts in all different shapes, sizes, and colors. The vast majority of us only eat a handful of these varieties. So you might be wondering which one is the healthiest. Walnuts appear to edge out the others. They contain some of the highest antioxidant and omega-3 fatty acid levels, particularly alpha-linolenic acid, which is found only in plants. In lab studies, walnuts beat out other nuts when it comes to suppressing cancer cell growth.

Almonds are popular for good reasons. Not only is their taste widely appealing, but they are also full of nutrients. Every ounce (approximately 23 almonds) is loaded with 6 grams of protein,

4 grams of fiber, as well as vitamin B2 (riboflavin), vitamin E, calcium, magnesium, and potassium.

Pecans are more than just a southern favorite. They not only complement many dishes easily, but are packed with nutrients containing more than twenty vitamins and minerals—including vitamin A, vitamin B9, vitamin E, calcium, magnesium, phosphorus, potassium, and zinc. Every ounce contains almost 3 grams of protein and 3 grams of fiber.

The oils made from nuts are healthy and convenient for cooking. Almond, hazelnut, macadamia, peanut, pecan, pistachio, and walnut are some of the varieties. Each has its own flavor, and they are prone to spoil faster than other oils. The key, however, is that they predominantly contain the heart-friendly unsaturated fats, unlike coconut oil, which is thought by so many to be healthy but is full of saturated fats—the type we want to consume in very low quantities.

Nuts and seeds and their oils are some of the most useful items you can have on your Clean 20 list. They can be eaten alone as a snack or added to all types of dishes and preparations, whether it's a salad, soup, or breakfast cereal. They are extremely portable, easy to store, and widely accessible. Make sure you choose raw nuts that haven't been processed with sugar or artificial ingredients. Some might be lightly salted, and that is fine if you look at the back of the label to make sure sodium levels are less than 140 milligrams per serving.

NUTS and SEEDS BENEFITS

- Good source of protein and fiber.
- Contain l-arginine, which might help improve blood vessel health.
- Contain several vitamins, including A, B-complex, and E.
- Contain heart-protective omega-3 fatty acids.
- Help lower LDL ("bad") cholesterol levels.
- Great snack to reduce hunger without artificial ingredients.
- Very easy to find and portable.

SHOPPING/HANDLING

- Roasted nuts are typically heavily salted, so look for unsalted or lightly salted varieties to avoid high sodium content.
- Nuts in their shells will keep for 6 to 12 months in a cool, dry place.
- Nut butters keep better in the refrigerator; if they separate, just mix.
- A natural nut butter *will* separate, but a creamy shelf-stable nut butter could be a signal that sugar and other additives have been used.
- Shop in the bulk bins, as the nuts and seeds stored there move quickly, thus are more likely to be fresher.
- Roast your own nuts in a pan at 275 to 300°F.

11 OATMEAL

More than just the stuff that was believed to "stick to your ribs," oatmeal is one of the healthiest grains on the planet. Our grandmothers weren't too far off when they insisted on feeding us a bowl of hearty oats before we marched off into a nippy fall or winter morning. Oatmeal contains soluble fiber, which doesn't actually stick to your ribs, but does stick around in your stomach longer, thus making you feel full longer. The benefits of this fiber are completely available in less than a cup of oatmeal.

In its early days, oatmeal was used to feed not only humans, but animals as well. In the early 1600s, European settlers brought oats to North America; they were featured in traditional porridges, puddings, and an assortment of baked goods, and were used as feed for horses.

Oatmeal is so healthy because it is truly a whole grain, meaning it contains all three parts of the grain (bran, endosperm, germ) that exist in nature. It is full of nutrients, including fiber, protein, vitamin B1, vitamin B7 (biotin), copper, iron, magnesium, manganese, phosphorous, and zinc. The less the oat is processed, the higher the amount of protein it will contain. Steel-cut oats have 7 grams of protein per ¼ cup (uncooked) serving, while rolled oats (more processed) have 3 grams per ¼ cup (uncooked) serving. For each ¼ cup serving the amount of fiber ranges from 2 to 4 grams depending on the type of oats used.

It might get confusing to figure out which oats you should buy since there are so many of them on the shelf. Here is a quick guide. Note that while these oats vary in their shape, texture, and cooking time, they are all still whole oats and their nutrition stays relatively the same except for small differences in fiber and protein content.

Whole oat groats: This is the most intact form of oat. The outer inedible hull of the grain kernel is removed and the groat is what is left. These take the longest time to cook and can't often be found in regular grocery stores. Most commonly you can purchase them in health food stores, but the vast majority of recipes do not use this type of oat.

Steel-cut oats (Irish oats): These are created when the whole groat is processed by using a sharp metal blade to chop groats into several pieces. (Note that it is not rolled, but chopped.) These oats look like rice that has been cut into pieces. They cook quicker than oat groats because water can more easily penetrate the smaller pieces. However, they could still take up to 20 to 30 minutes to cook and require some stirring. This is probably longer than what most are accustomed to when cooking oatmeal.

Scottish oats: These are very similar to the steel-cut oats, but rather than being cut by a steel blade, they are ground into bits and pieces by a stone-grinding process. Cooking time is about the same as for steel-cut oats, but the porridge it creates tends to be creamier.

Rolled oats (regular, also known as old-fashioned): These are created when oat groats are steamed and then rolled into flakes. They are flat, irregularly round, and slightly textured. They cook faster than steel-cut oats because there is more surface area. They can absorb more liquid, and can hold their shape throughout the cooking process.

Rolled oats (quick or instant): These are the most processed of the three major oat varieties. They are created by being precooked, dried, and then rolled and pressed to the extent that they are even thinner than regular rolled oats.

Oatmeal is a versatile grain that can be used in a variety of preparations. Boil it for a breakfast cereal, add it to a smoothie, bake it inside an apple (see recipe, page 177), or make it an ingredient in your homemade cookies. There are plenty of breakfast, lunch, and snack recipes that you can find to make good use of this healthy, sturdy grain.

OATS BENEFITS

- High in fiber (particularly beta-glucan).
- Source of manganese, selenium, phosphorous, and magnesium.
- Rich in vitamin E.
- Source of antioxidants.
- Lower bad cholesterol.
- Help control blood pressure.
- May reduce type 2 diabetes risk.
- Helps reduce risk of coronary artery disease.
- Lower risk of colorectal cancer.

SHOPPING/HANDLING

- Choose an oat that dovetails with the amount of time you have to cook it.
- Add to batter or dough for muffins and breads.
- For a creamier cereal preparation, use milk instead of water.
- Substitute for white bread crumbs in recipes.
- Store in an airtight container in a dry, dark, cool place.

12 QUINOA

Quinoa is an edible seed of a plant from the Amaranthaceae family—*Chenopodium quinoa*. It dates back thousands of years, with some estimates placing its popularity all the way back to 3000 B.C. in the Andes mountain regions of South America. Quinoa was a staple food during the Incan Empire, largely because of its

ability to survive a variety of weather conditions. Sun, little rain-
fall, high altitudes, subfreezing temperatures, bad soil—the
ever-durable quinoa plant can withstand it all.

As a matter of convenience and tradition, quinoa has largely
been classified as a grain, similar to the classification of rice, wheat,
oats, cornmeal, corn (maize), barley, and others. These are also
called cereal grasses—grasses whose starchy grains are used as
food. Botanically, however, quinoa is not a true grain or cereal
grass. It actually belongs to a subclassification of plants that is
very different from grass. In fact, researchers call it a "pseudo-
cereal" because even though it's not a true cereal grass, it can still
be easily ground into flour just like grains. Another reason quinoa is typically classified with cereal grasses is because it tends
to be prepared and consumed in a similar fashion. It has a
crunchy texture and nutty flavor and is gluten-free, which is
important for those with a sensitivity to gluten or wheat.

Quinoa is a nutritional powerhouse and is considered by many
to be a superfood. It contains high levels of fiber, protein, manganese, copper, phosphorous, magnesium, and B-vitamins. And
that's just the beginning. It also serves up folate, iron, zinc, calcium, vitamin E, antioxidants, and heart-healthy fats such as
omega-3 fatty acids and the monounsaturated fat oleic acid. Its
nutrient richness is highlighted by the amount and quality of
its protein—a nutritional shortcoming for many grains. Quinoa
contains complete protein, which means it contains all nine of
the essential amino acids—amino acids that can't be made by the
body, but must come from food. There are relatively few foods
that contain complete protein, as most foods typically lack one
or more of the essential amino acids. Quinoa has an important

high protein-to-carbohydrate ratio when compared to grain products and was deemed so beneficial that NASA proposed it as an ideal food for long-duration space fights. The quality of its protein is similar to the well-regarded casein protein found in milk.

Quinoa is also considered to be a whole grain from a nutritional standpoint, because the entire grain seed is intact and none of the three integral parts are removed. When whole grains are refined, processed, or milled, that means that one or more of the three parts have been removed or altered, and unfortunately this removes important nutrients and decreases the nutritional value.

While there are hundreds of types of quinoa, the most common found in stores are white, also called ivory quinoa, and red. Experts note that there is little nutritional difference between the two; however, there is a difference when it comes to cooking them. White quinoa is the mildest and least crunchy and cooks the fastest. Black quinoa is much crunchier and takes much longer to cook. Red quinoa exists somewhere in the middle.

Quinoa has many proposed health benefits, including reducing the risk of type 2 diabetes, cardiovascular disease, obesity, colon cancer, and high blood pressure. The antioxidant flavonoids quercetin and kaempferol are abundantly found in quinoa and are believed to be helpful in staving off some of these diseases. Quinoa is full of anti-inflammatory nutrients. In fact, some animal studies have looked at these anti-inflammatory effects and they appear to be promising, potentially leading to lower levels of inflammation in fat tissue and in the lining of the intestine. Taking into account all that quinoa has to offer, it's a sure bet to include in the Clean 20.

QUINOA BENEFITS

- Source of fiber and protein; also source of copper, folate, iron, magnesium, manganese, phosphorus, and zinc.
- Contains quercetin—a powerful polyphenol antioxidant.
- Helps lower blood sugar levels.
- Gluten free.

SHOPPING/HANDLING

- If you plan to use the seed in baking, use quinoa flour or flakes.
- White quinoa cooks the fastest and has the mildest flavor.
- Avoid cooking in microwave, as it's difficult to cook consistently.
- Try to buy prerinsed to save yourself some effort and time.
- Rinse yourself even if prerinsed to make sure all the saponins (compounds found on the outer surface that form a waxy protective coating) are off.
- When cooking, use 2 cups water to 1 cup quinoa, boil, then simmer.

13 SEAFOOD *(OPTIONS: COD, CRAB, HALIBUT, LOBSTER, OYSTERS, SALMON, SEA BASS, SHRIMP, TUNA)*

When it comes to naming some of the healthiest foods on the planet, there's no need to argue when it comes to seafood, particularly fish. Full of protein, vitamin D, vitamin B2, calcium, phosphorous, iron, zinc, iodine, potassium, omega-3 fatty acids, and other nutrients, fish loads up our health bucket at relatively little financial and calorie cost. How health-boosting is fish? The American Heart Association recommends eating it at least two times per week. It can lower blood pressure, reduce the risk of heart attack or stroke, and keep our brains healthy.

Omega-3 fatty acids are critical, and two types of them are found in fish—EPA (eicosapentaenoic acid) and DHA (docosahexaenoic acid). Omega-3 fatty acids are found in every kind of fish, but there are particularly high levels in the fatty fish such as salmon, tuna, herring, sardines, trout, and oysters. Our bodies can produce omega-3 fatty acids, but not enough to satisfy our needs, so we have to get them in our food.

While there are too many fish to review, there are five very popular fish that not only reign gastronomically for many, but also pack a good dose of nutrition. They are:

Salmon: One of the most healthful fish in the world, largely inhabiting the northern Atlantic and Pacific oceans. Full of vitamin B12, vitamin D, selenium, vitamin B3, omega-3 fats, protein, phosphorus, and vitamin B6. Flavorful, fatty, and flaky, this fish is one of the most popular in the world and can be found almost anywhere fish are sold. While there are many varieties of salmon, it's important to note that all of them are full of health-promoting nutrients that can help prevent disease, improve lean muscle mass, and boost the immune system.

Sea bass: Ranked alongside salmon as one of the most popular fish in the world. This lean saltwater fish is meaty and can be cooked in a variety of ways. The different types of sea bass have different flavor profiles, but they all generally have lean meat that is moderately firm, flakes into small to medium pieces, and has a delicate flavor. "Sea bass" is a generic term that's used for different fish from various species, and technically most are not even bass. Some of the more common include: black, blue spotted (actually a grouper), Chilean (actually a Patagonian toothfish), European, giant (actually a grouper), and white (actually a croaker). Sea bass offers a variety of nutrients, most notably protein, vitamin D, vitamin B6, phosphorous, selenium, and magnesium.

Halibut: A lean fish with mild, sweet-tasting white flesh. It tends to have large flakes, its meat is firm, and the texture is tender. Typically found on the Pacific Coast from northern California to the Bering Sea and from the Sea of Japan to Russia, halibut tend to spend most of their time on the bottom of the ocean in deeper waters. Some of the varieties include Atlantic, California, Greenland Turbot, and Pacific, most available at a typical grocery store. Low in saturated fat, halibut is a good source of protein, vitamin B3, vitamin B6, potassium, phosphorous, and selenium.

Tuna: One of the most versatile fish in the way that it's prepared and conveniently purchased, raw or canned. There are several varieties that include albacore, yellowfin, blackfin, bluefin, and skipjack. Tuna is full of nutrients, including selenium, vitamin B3, vitamin B12, vitamin B6, vitamin D, protein, phosphorous, potassium, and iodine. The most common canned fish, tuna is widely available throughout the entire year. "White" tuna is albacore. "Light" tuna varieties include skipjack, yellowfin, bigeye, or a combination of the three. White tuna has almost triple the healthy omega-3 fatty acids, but be careful, as it has nearly triple the levels of mercury. Tuna packed in water or vegetable broth or "natural juices" has fewer calories than oil-packed and is milder in flavor.

Cod: A fan favorite, cod is a staple in restaurants that offer seafood and is available throughout the year, making it extremely convenient, accessible, and relatively inexpensive. It thrives in the Pacific and North Atlantic Oceans and delivers a mild-flavored flesh that can be a great substitute for those looking to get protein without consuming red meat. It can be effectively cooked in the oven, on top of the stove, or on a grill, and its mild flavor makes it accommodating to spices and other ingredients that it's cooked with and other foods on the plate. Cod is often fried, and if you've had the classic fish and chips made famous by the English working class, then you've been treated to cod's most popular preparation. Beyond its great taste, cod boasts a respectable nutrition profile that includes protein, vitamin B12, vitamin B3, vitamin B6, iodine, selenium, phosphorous, choline, and some omega-3 fats (not as much as some of the other fish).

Recognizing and purchasing fresh fish can be an art in and of itself, but it's important to understand some of the basics. If you're buying a whole fish, start with the eyes and make sure they are bright and clear. Fish eyes fade the older they get, so a dull-eyed fish is likely past its prime. Whether it's a whole fish or a fillet, you want the body of your fish to be shiny or have a metallic appearance. Avoid those that have dulled or have discolored patches. The gills of a fish can say a lot. Make sure they're a healthy, vibrant red. Last, smell the fish. If it actually smells "fishy," that's a problem, and you shouldn't purchase it. A fresh fish should smell like clean water.

Buying a fish fillet is a little different. Touch the flesh and it should spring back. The color should be even in tone, with no areas of severe discoloration. Sniff it and make sure it doesn't smell fishy—a salty or seaweed aroma is perfectly acceptable. Don't be afraid to ask the fishmonger when the fish was brought in. Make sure the fish is in a display that is well kempt and heavily iced.

There has been a lot of debate about which is the best fish to buy with regards to how it was raised and caught. There could be an entire book dedicated to this topic, so I will try to give you a very succinct guide to follow.

1. Wild-caught fish is always best. The fish has been allowed to live and swim in its natural environment without major intrusion. If it doesn't mention the living conditions of the fish on the package, ask the fishmonger.

2. Farm-raised is less desirable than wild and is the next most common condition, but even this is broken down into categories.

    a. Tanks or cages: Fish are held captive in a large area and are not allowed to swim free. They are sometimes fed an unhealthy diet that might include hormones.

    b. Open-water cages or nets: Fish are in a captive environment, but the holding area is in an open-water system that flows freely through the cage or net, thus allowing wastes and contamination to flow freely out of the direct environment of the fish.

3. Make sure labeling of the farm-raised fish says that it's without antibiotics or hormones; farmed in low-density (not cramped)

pens or tanks; the fish were fed a more natural diet; and there was no treatment with synthetic herbicides.

4. General rule of thumb: if you don't understand the label, ask your fishmonger the questions above.

SEAFOOD BENEFITS

- Rich source of protein.
- Rich source of omega-3 fatty acids.
- Rich source of vitamin D.
- Good source of vitamin A.
- Potentially helps lower risk of heart attacks and strokes.
- Protects brain from age-related deterioration.
- Improves condition of skin and hair.
- Low calorie to nutrient ratio.

SHOPPING/HANDLING

- Choose "wild-caught" fish as the best option.
- Look for pole-caught or line-caught fish.
- Farmed-raised fish is less desirable, but choose "Responsibly Farm Raised."
- Choose fish displayed well and surrounded by an abundance of clean crushed ice.
- If storing before cooking, wrap well in plastic, then place in airtight bag.
- Whole fish can be refrigerated for up to 2 days; fillets and steaks 1 to 2 days.
- Be careful when cooking frozen fish, as it can easily overcook.
- Consider canned fish, but make sure it's "wild" or "pole-caught" or "line-caught."

One caveat about fish and mercury. Some fish are high in mercury, and if enough accumulates in your body, this can be dangerous to your nervous system. But this by no means is a suggestion that you should avoid fish, but rather that you should make smart choices. In fact, according to the Department of Agriculture's Dietary Guidelines for Americans, issued in 2015, "for the majority of wild-caught and farmed species, neither the risks of mercury nor organic pollutants outweigh the health benefits of seafood consumption." Take a look at the table below to get a better understanding of the mercury content of certain fish. The FDA and EPA say that most women and young children should avoid the first four of the highest-mercury fish. Everyone else should consume less than 24 ounces per week, an amount that the vast majority of people don't eat anyway.

LOWEST MERCURY FISH

Shrimp, scallops, sardines, wild and Alaska salmon, oysters, squid, tilapia.

LOW MERCURY

Atlantic croaker, Atlantic mackerel, catfish, cod, crab, crawfish, flounder and sole (flatfish), haddock, mullet, pollock, trout, canned light tuna.

HIGHER MERCURY

Grouper, Chilean sea bass, bluefish, halibut, sablefish (black cod), Spanish mackerel, fresh tuna (except skipjack), canned white (albacore) tuna.

HIGHEST MERCURY

Swordfish, shark, king mackerel, Gulf tilefish, marlin, orange roughy.

14 SQUASH *(BASKET BUDDIES: CARROTS, CUCUMBERS, EGGPLANT, PARSNIPS, ZUCCHINI)*

Squash are easily recognized gourds dating back some ten thousand years to Mesoamerica. Famous for being one of the "three sisters" crops (corn, beans, and squash) cultivated by Native Americans, they were a staple food of the early American diet. They belong to the same family that includes melons and cucumbers. "Squash" is actually a rather broad term that encompasses a number of different types of what we call vegetables (though botanically speaking they are fruits) such as zucchini and pumpkins. One of the most versatile vegetables available throughout the world, it serves not only great flavor, but a respectable amount of health-boosting nutrition.

There are several varieties of squash to choose from, but the two major groups are divided between summer squash and winter squash. They earned their names long ago when each variety could only grow during that time of the year. Now, both varieties are available year-round. The major difference between the two is that summer squash are picked while still young and tender, while winter squash are not harvested until later when they mature. Summer squash has a soft shell with tender, light-colored flesh. Winter squash has a harder, more rigid shell with dark, tougher flesh and seeds. Summer squash must be eaten or processed fairly quickly, which is why it's often included in breads or soup, or steamed or sautéed. Winter squash can be stored for months in the right conditions and is often pureed into soups, baked, or sautéed.

One of the great things about summer squash is that it's mostly water, which means it packs in relatively few calories. Easy to cook, it has a mild taste and willingly takes on the flavor of the oils and spices of foods that are cooked with it.

There are several varieties of summer squash, and they include zucchini, yellow crookneck, yellow straightneck, and scallop. Some of the common winter squash varieties include butternut, acorn, Hubbard, turban, and kabocha.

Squash is not the nutritional powerhouse some of the other ingredients on our list are, but it is still a great addition. Both summer and winter squashes contain a broad spectrum of nutrients: vitamin C, vitamin B6, vitamin K, vitamin A, copper, manganese, magnesium, and folate. It also contains fiber, which helps with everything from reducing digestive problems to preventing heart disease by lowering cholesterol levels. This makes it a very good partner with the other health-boosting foods populating our list. Another reason why it makes the cut: it's particularly low in calories for all that it delivers. Summer squash only serves up 36 calories for a cup of cooked slices, while winter squash clocks in at around 76 calories per cup.

Squash is a largely underrated food ingredient, but many chefs will tell you how easy it is to work with and how great a guest it can be to the other foods that are being prepared. Squash can be sautéed, baked, grilled, roasted, pureed, boiled and mashed, and steamed. It can complement almost any dish and can even stand alone, depending on your choice of preparation. A little bit of olive oil and some spices can turn this gourd into something that's great!

SQUASH BENEFITS

- Very high nutrition-to-calorie ratio.
- Improves cardiovascular health through magnesium and potassium.
- Improves lung health through its high vitamin A content.
- Boosts immune system through antioxidants and vitamins.
- Helps regulate blood sugars through fiber and B-complex vitamins.
- Anti-inflammatory properties due to omega-3 fatty acids and carotenoids.

SHOPPING/HANDLING

- For summer squash, look for smaller fruits with bright skin and no discoloration/damage.
- Summer squash taste best when small- to medium-sized (7 inches or less).
- Squash should be plump and stem ends fresh and green.
- Winter squash should feel heavy for its size.
- Winter squash are best when stems are attached and are rounded and dry, not blackened or collapsed.
- Choose winter squash that is rich and deep in color.
- Winter squash skin should be dull and matte (if shiny, it was picked too early).
- Store summer squash in the refrigerator in the crisper drawer, not a plastic bag.
- Store winter squash in a cool, dry place for up to 3 months.
- Once chopped, squash can be refrigerated for up to 7 days.

15 SWEET POTATOES

While these orange root vegetables are often admired for their contributions to delicious pies, they offer a lot more in the form of action-packed nutrition. Believed to have originated in Central and South America thousands of years ago, they grow almost like a vine with white flowers. The part that we eat is the root of the plant.

There are many varieties of sweet potatoes besides the popular orange. They can be found in yellow, white, purple, and pink. According to the Cleveland Clinic, the purple variety is a great way to load up on disease-fighting antioxidants. The orange and yellow varieties contain the most vitamin A.

Sweet potatoes tend to be more nutritious than white potatoes. Not only are they full of vitamins (particularly A, B, and C), but they have a lower glycemic index (GI), which means they don't raise blood sugar levels in the body as fast. This is largely due to all of the manganese sweet potatoes contain and how manganese helps the body process carbohydrates. Sweet potatoes are largely fat-free just like their paler siblings, but contain fewer calories. In addition to their antioxidants, they have anti-inflammatory properties that can be beneficial to overall health.

There has been some confusion about the differences between sweet potatoes and yams. While the two look and sometimes taste alike, they are very different plants. Yams are never orange, but typically white-fleshed and sometimes purple. Yams tend to have rough, dark skin that appears to be hairy. They are starchy and much drier than sweet potatoes and are definitely not as sweet. Sweet potatoes are often erroneously marked as yams, but in the vast majority of cases the vegetables labeled "yams" are actually sweet potatoes. The orange flesh is distinctive of sweet potatoes and their skin tends to be smoother, and often has a reddish-brown hue.

Sweet potatoes are simple to cook and can be prepared in a variety of ways. Boiling and baking them tend to be the most common preparations. They can be mashed, quartered and baked, fried, or added to casseroles and desserts. (see Baked Sweet Potato Fries recipe, page 205). You don't have to be a trained chef to cook many exciting dishes with sweet potatoes, as the recipes tend to include few ingredients and require little work.

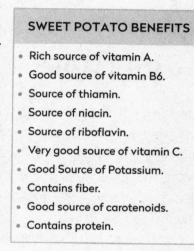

SWEET POTATO BENEFITS

- Rich source of vitamin A.
- Good source of vitamin B6.
- Source of thiamin.
- Source of niacin.
- Source of riboflavin.
- Very good source of vitamin C.
- Good Source of Potassium.
- Contains fiber.
- Good source of carotenoids.
- Contains protein.

SHOPPING/HANDLING

- Make sure they are heavy for their size.
- Choose those without mold, blemishes, or sprouts.
- Skin should be taut and not wrinkled.
- Make sure they are firm.
- They should be stored in a cool, dry place, but *not* refrigerated.

In a side-by-side comparison, the results are mixed with respect to whether sweet potatoes or yams are healthiest. Sweet potatoes are lower in calories—76 calories for half a cup, compared to yams, which have 116. Sweet potatoes have fewer carbs, but yams have less sugar. Yams have about 25% more fiber and a little more protein. They also have more potassium. Sweet potatoes, however, have a lot more vitamin A. Both sweet potatoes and yams are nutritious, so you can't go wrong with either choice.

16 TOMATOES

These juicy bulbous fruits—yes, tomatoes are a fruit and not a vegetable—are a true superfood and integral to a variety of cuisines around the globe. Easy to cultivate and quick to grow, they are an inexpensive and reliable food source. Their color is a great indication of how packed they are with great nutritional value.

The array of nutrients tomatoes contain is nothing short of staggering. They boast an impressive amount of vitamins A, C, and K as well as substantial amounts of vitamins B1, B6, and B9. If that weren't enough, they are full of fiber and protein as well as potassium, copper, vitamin B3, magnesium, phosphorous, manganese, and chromium. Some of their most showcased health powers lie in their quad of antioxidants that are thought to help prevent disease—alpha and beta-carotene, lutein, and lycopene.

Carotenoids are the orange, yellow, and red-pigmented compounds that can't be synthesized by humans and are only available through diet. These compounds are beneficial to our health, helpful for protecting vision and fighting damage to our cells. There are more than 750 naturally occurring carotenoids in nature, and tomatoes contain four of the most effective of them—lycopene, beta-carotene, lutein, and zeaxanthin. Beta-carotene is a well-researched antioxidant that is converted into vitamin A (retinol), crucial for healthy skin, vision, mucus membranes, and our immune system.

Lycopene has gotten a lot of attention lately and has undergone extensive research in regard to its health benefits. It is a carotenoid and thought to have the highest antioxidant activity in its class. Lycopene is believed to help prevent prostate cancer, and some researchers have reported its potential to help reduce the risk of pancreatic cancer. One study found that when tomatoes were eaten along with healthier fats such as olive or avocado oil, the body's absorption of lycopene more than doubled.

TOMATO BENEFITS

- Rich source of vitamins, minerals, and antioxidants.
- Defends against and fights prostate, cervical, stomach, and rectal cancers.
- Reduces LDL (bad) cholesterol levels.
- Reduces heart disease risk.

SHOPPING/HANDLING

- Tomatoes' phytonutrients become more concentrated and bioavailable when cooked into a sauce or paste.
- Don't buy tomatoes from a refrigerated case.
- Keep tomatoes out at room temperature.
- Try to buy tomatoes loosely displayed rather than boxed so you can evaluate them better.
- Choose plump, heavy tomatoes with smooth skins free of cracks or bruises.
- The tomatoes should smell fresh with a bit of earthiness.
- Only buy fully ripe tomatoes if you plan to use them immediately. Ripe tomatoes are soft and yield to pressure.

17 TURKEY

There's nothing more synonymous with Thanksgiving than a plump, stuffed turkey sitting in the middle of a busy table. While turkey is the centerpiece of our holiday feast, it is a great choice of meat any time of the year. Moist, full of protein (second in quantity to beef and equal to chicken), vitamins, and minerals, turkey delivers in so many ways.

Turkey provides a robust concoction of nutrients, including the vitamins niacin, B5, B6, B12, and riboflavin. You will also get the minerals iron, phosphorous, potassium, zinc, and selenium. Selenium is noteworthy because not only is it available in large amounts, but it's essential for proper thyroid and immune function.

There are two types of turkey meat—the breast and dark meat. Taste and color are not the only differences between the two. The light meat of the breast contains fewer calories, less fat, and more protein. The dark meat, however, contains slightly more vitamins and minerals. In either case, avoid the skin when possible, as it contains a substantial amount of fat and dramatically increases the calorie count when consumed.

Turkey is a great choice whether it's used as lunch meat, in a casserole, or simply sliced for dinner. It can be purchased in ground form and molded into meatballs, sausage, or burgers. Try to buy fresh turkey whenever possible, as processed turkey in deli meats, hot dogs, and bacon can be high in sodium. If purchasing frozen, prepackaged turkey burgers, make sure you look at the nutrition label, as they can be full of added salt and other preservatives. Many think that because a product is made of turkey it's automatically healthier. Not so. Manufacturers still add all kinds of other ingredients that can increase the fat content, calories, and sodium. This is why reading the label is always critical when trying to make a healthier decision.

Setting the record straight, turkey is not the reason why you're falling asleep after that hefty Thanksgiving dinner. Tryptophan found in the meat has been fingered as the culprit. This amino acid is the precursor to the brain chemical serotonin that's associated with relaxation and sleep. However, the amount of tryptophan in a single serving of turkey is not enough to make you drowsy. In fact, almost all meats contain some level of tryptophan.

TURKEY BENEFITS

- High in protein.
- Low in fat.
- Rich in selenium.
- Source of vitamins B5, B6, and B12.
- Source of niacin.
- Source of choline, phosphorous, and zinc.

SHOPPING/HANDLING

- For the healthiest, buy organic or pasture-raised.
- Look for meat that is supple.
- Make sure you cook it all the way through (165 degrees).
- Uncooked refrigerated turkey lasts 2 to 3 days.
- Cooked turkey lasts 4 to 5 days in the refrigerator.
- If purchasing processed meat, look at the sodium level.

18 WHOLE-GRAIN BREAD
(OPTIONS: SPROUTED GRAIN, SPELT)

For many it seems almost impossible to live without bread. In some form it tends to be a part of almost every meal we consume. Bread would never be classified as a superfood, but it does have a decent amount of nutritional value. This, of course, depends on the type of bread that you choose. To make matters simple, for the next twenty days you will only be concerned with two types of bread—100% whole wheat and 100% whole grain. White bread, along with white flour, is completely off the menu.

Bread is actually a relatively simple creation that comes from flour. If it's white bread, then white flour is used. If it's whole-grain bread, then whole-grain flour is used. Both white and whole-grain flours come from the same original source—the whole-grain wheat kernel. The difference, however, is in the processing. The white flour is stripped of two of the three parts of the grain—bran (grain's outer layer) and germ (sprouting section of the seed)—two parts that provide vitamin E, protein, B vitamins, antioxidants, healthy fats, and fiber. The kernel is smashed in the process and eventually milled and bleached so that it appears white.

Whole-grain flour also undergoes processing, but all three parts of the grain are included. (See the section on oatmeal, page 44.) This is why you must purchase bread that says either 100% whole grain or 100% whole wheat. The "100%" tells you that all the grains in the bread are whole. If the packaging says "Whole Grain," all that's really telling you is that the bread contains some whole grains in it, but not all of the grains are whole. It could also contain refined grains along with those whole grains.

Even the 100% whole-grain and 100% whole-wheat breads that you typically see in the grocery store can contain added sugar. If you look at the nutritional label, you will see sugar near the top of the ingredients list. For these twenty days, you are trying to stay away from added sugars, so this is where it can get tricky. Do your best to find breads that don't have added sugars. This might not be easy, but there are specialty stores that sell whole-grain and whole-wheat breads with very low sugar—1 to 3 grams. If you simply don't have access to these low-sugar breads in the stores you frequent, or because you're traveling, then the popular bread brands that have more sugar will be allowed. Also, you can buy more than just a loaf of sliced bread. There's pita, sourdough, breadcrumbs, and English muffins. Be careful of purchasing a bread just based on its color, as the brown color you're seeing might simply be sugars or molasses added during the manufacturing process. Manufacturers know that many people assume brown bread is synonymous with being healthy, so they add all of these artificial ingredients and market it as healthy. Rye bread is the star of this confusion. Look at the first ingredient listed on the packaging. Typically, it says "unbleached enriched flour." You still need to see that "100%" demarcation even with a dark, healthy-looking bread like rye.

The nomenclature can also be misleading. Just because it says multigrain or seven-grain doesn't mean that it is completely whole-grain bread. "Multi" means "many," so all that labeling means is that there are many grains in that bread. That doesn't mean the grains haven't been processed and refined. Same for the seven-grain label. All that tells you is that there are seven grains within the bread. Big deal. It says nothing about whether the grains are whole or refined.

WHOLE-GRAIN BREAD BENEFITS

- Offers all the health benefits of whole grains (see Oatmeal, page 44).
- Promotes healthy bowel function.
- Helps maintain a healthy weight.
- Helps lower risk for heart disease.
- Absorbed more slowly than breads made from refined or enriched flour.

SHOPPING/HANDLING

- Make sure the label says 100% whole grain or 100% whole wheat.
- Read packaging label to make sure there's no added sugar or artificial ingredients.
- Make sure whole grain or whole wheat is the first ingredient in the packaging ingredient list.
- Rye bread is usually not a 100% whole-grain bread.
- "100% natural" label means nothing; don't be fooled.

19 WHOLE-WHEAT PASTA

White pasta has been so ingrained in our gastronomic consciousness that the thought of cooking brown pasta and serving it with meatballs and marinara sauce was tantamount to sacrilege. But minds and palates have opened, and whole-wheat pasta offerings have increased on store shelves for good reasons. Whole-wheat pasta is healthier, and when you prepare it with sauces and spices, you really can't taste the difference between the white and whole-wheat noodles.

The major difference between white and whole-wheat pasta really lies in how the noodles are processed or manufactured. The whole wheat contains the three nutrient-rich parts of the grain (bran, endosperm, and germ). White flour has gone through a refining process where the whole wheat kernel is stripped of the bran and germ, leaving just the endosperm. In some cases, manufacturers then add back some of the nutrients they stripped, such as iron and the B vitamins—hence the term you see on the package, "enriched." But even with these nutrients added back, the white pasta still falls far short of the whole-wheat pasta and the power of its unrefined whole grains. Retailers and manufacturers tend to like white pasta because it has a longer shelf life, which means less spoilage and more time to sell the product to consumers.

There are various types of whole-grain pastas that you can purchase. Barley, brown rice, buckwheat, corn, farro, kamut, millet, oats, quinoa, and spelt are some of the whole grains that are used to make pasta. Given the larger offerings, you can find these whole-grain pastas in various noodle shapes from bow-tie to spaghetti to fettuccine and rigatoni.

When shopping for whole-wheat or whole-grain pasta, don't just make a decision based on the color of the noodle. Seeing the brown color is a good place to start, but you should also look at the ingredients list and make sure the word "whole" appears in front of each grain that's listed. The terminology can be deceiving, so you must pay close attention. A label that says "multigrain" simply means that the pasta is made from more than one type of grain, but that doesn't mean the grains are whole. If it says "100 percent wheat," that means it contains only wheat flour, but it doesn't necessarily mean the flour is *whole* wheat. When you see "made with whole grains," all that is really telling you is that some of the flour used was whole-grain flour, but typically these products contain a higher proportion of refined flour.

There are many other terms you will see when purchasing whole-wheat pasta and you need to be mindful of them. Organic can be good, but it doesn't equal whole grain. Vegetable pastas can be good also, but it doesn't mean they are whole-grain pastas—you still have to read the label. One of the easiest ways to make sure you're getting the good stuff—look for the black-and-gold stamp from the nonprofit Whole Grains Council. One stamp means that it contains at least 8 grams of whole grains per serving, while the second stamp means that the product contains 100% whole grains—all the grains are whole and not refined.

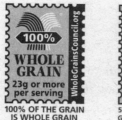
100% OF THE GRAIN
IS WHOLE GRAIN

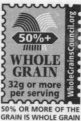
50% OR MORE OF THE
GRAIN IS WHOLE GRAIN

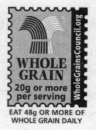
EAT 48g OR MORE OF
WHOLE GRAIN DAILY

WHOLE-WHEAT PASTA BENEFITS

- Contains all three nutrient-rich parts of the whole grain.
- High in B vitamins and minerals such as copper, magnesium, and manganese.
- Contains more fiber and protein than white pasta.
- Helps decrease risk of developing conditions that predispose to diabetes and heart disease.

SHOPPING/HANDLING

- Look for the word "whole" in front of the listed grains.
- Just because the brand name of the product sounds healthy doesn't mean it is—still read the label.
- Spinach and tomato pastas are not necessarily whole grain; must state that they are made with whole grains.
- Organic pastas are not always whole grain—read the label carefully.
- Look for the Whole Grains Council stamp.
- Cook 2 to 3 minutes longer than white pasta.

20 YOGURT

Almost every grocery store dairy section is dominated by a multitude of yogurt offerings. This is for good reason—yogurt is extremely healthy and tasty and a staple in most diets. Yogurt's main ingredient is milk, so its nutrient-rich profile makes a lot of sense. With each scoop, you can expect to get a dose of animal protein (approximately 9 grams per 6-ounce serving), calcium, vitamin B2, vitamin B12, magnesium, phosphorus, and potassium.

Many yogurt brands (not all) also contain probiotics—live bacteria that are considered to be friendly bacteria that have beneficial health effects when consumed. Our body's digestive system already contains hundreds of different types of bacteria that are important to maintain the health of our gut and assist in the proper functioning of the digestive process. Two of the main probiotics found in fermented milk products such as yogurt are lactic acid bacteria and bifidobacteria. If a yogurt is pasteurized (heat-treated), the probiotic bacteria are killed and thus don't provide any health benefits. Thus, if you're looking to take advantage of what probiotics can offer, you need to choose a yogurt that has "active" or "live" cultures. Beyond assisting with digestion, some of the probiotic health benefits include: lowering cholesterol levels, improving the ability to digest the milk sugar lactose, making vitamins, enhancing immunity, and reducing constipation.

Yogurt also has something called ruminant trans fats, also known as dairy trans fats. These are very different from the manufactured hydrogenated trans fats in processed foods that you should avoid at all costs. There are animal studies that show these natural dairy trans fats could have health benefits, but studies relating to humans so far are inconclusive.

There are so many brands and preparations of yogurt on the shelves that it can be difficult to tell which is healthiest. The answer isn't as straightforward as one might like. It really depends on what you're looking for. One of the biggest places to start is Greek vs. regular yogurt. If looking at an overall score, Greek yogurt is the victor. In general, it has less cholesterol, less sugar, lower carbohydrate count, more protein, and less sodium. Low-fat or fat-free yogurt typically has less fat and more calcium, and while it has more cholesterol than Greek yogurt, the amount it contains is still considered to be very low.

Sugar can be a problem with many of the yogurt brands and it's something you should consider. Some yogurts can have a whopping 30 grams of sugar per serving, which means more than 7 teaspoons of sugar! There are plenty of brands that offer products with low sugar and low sodium, yet contain substantial quantities of protein and calcium. Take your time in the dairy section and decide which nutrition profile and flavor work best for you, then go for it.

YOGURT BENEFITS

- Inexpensive source of protein and calcium.
- Yogurt with active probiotics can help the digestive system and boost immune system.
- May help prevent osteoporosis (thinning of the bones).
- May reduce risk of high blood pressure.
- Widely available and extremely portable.
- Increases your feeling of fullness.

SHOPPING/HANDLING

- Choose low-fat or fat-free to be conscious of calories.
- Make sure the sugar content is less than 10 grams.
- Purchase yogurt without "fruit on the bottom" to reduce the sugar content, and add your own fresh fruit.
- Look at the nutrition label and choose a yogurt that has vitamin D.
- To get the benefits of probiotics, look for the label that says "live" cultures or "active" cultures or both.
- Add ½ teaspoon ground flaxseed to your yogurt and get almost 3 grams of fiber and 2 grams of healthy omega-3s.
- Add to a smoothie to make it creamier.
- A convenient and rich snack when eaten with fresh fruit to get fiber and protein at once.

Part II

The Plan

three

The Clean 20 Rules

I have designed the Clean 20 to be as accessible and versatile as possible. I don't expect you to go to a grocery store and empty your bank account in order to find the items on the list. I don't expect you to be locked into your house for the next twenty days so that you are in complete control of your food environment and all the ingredients that go into your food. You will be at work or at a restaurant or in an airport and you still need to eat and not feel like you're a criminal because you might have to slightly alter the plan. Remember, the purpose of the Clean 20 is to reintroduce your body to the wonders of clean eating and to give your organs a break from all the processed foods that dominate the choices in our stores and restaurants.

Clean food and clean recipes don't have to be boring or flavorless, despite the image conjured of plain chicken and bland raw vegetables. In fact, clean foods can be just as tasty and exciting as those processed foods that are loaded with lots of additives and artificial flavor enhancers. Spices and clean condiments can go a long way to liven up recipes and thrill your palate. We have grown so accustomed to processed foods that we need to be reacquainted with the authentic flavors of real, natural food. So take your time with the ingredients. Taste them raw or with spices—something that will happen over the next twenty days.

I don't like rules. I think the mere mention of the word inspires eye-rolling and rebellion and annoyance. Most people don't like to be told what they can and can't do as well as what they can and can't eat. But in order for you to maximize your results and reset your experience for the next twenty days, I created guidelines that will give you the greatest chance of success and keep you most in line with the plan's overall mission.

I have learned over the years that no chapter or book can answer all of the possible questions that come up. Just when you think you've covered all the bases, someone finds a topic or angle that hasn't been addressed. I am not perfect, and this plan is not perfect. However, between the guidelines below and some common sense, the next twenty days should work well for you.

The key to success on this plan definitely lies in the departments of planning and preparation. Take a little time and think about what the next several days will look like: what meals you'll be consuming and where they'll be consumed. If you're going to be traveling, take that into account and think about what foods will most likely be available to you while on the road. Plan accordingly.

1. Dairy is good

Dairy has been getting beaten up lately, and I think it's simply unfair. Sometimes dieting trends simply become too trendy for our own good. The wave of no-dairy sentiment is largely misplaced and for many people can be dangerous, as dairy provides nutrients that are critical to our overall health. Calcium, potassium, vitamin D, and protein are chief among these nutrients. Dairy is the primary source of calcium in our diets and is needed to build and preserve strong bones as well as teeth. Potassium is essential to life. Every time your heart beats it relies on potassium, which helps trigger the heart to pump and squeeze blood through the body. Potassium is also critical in helping our muscles move, nerves conduct electricity, kidneys filter blood, and blood vessels maintain blood pressure. Vitamin D works to maintain proper levels of phosphorous and calcium in the body: that's why it's an important component in building and maintaining healthy bones and teeth. It also plays a role in muscle function and keeping our immune system healthy. Dairy products such as yogurt, milk, and cheese (a great source of calcium, vitamin B12, and sodium) are rich in so many nutrients that make and keep us healthy. Some may have an intolerance to lactose—the sugar found in milk and other dairy products—and need to be careful of which products they consume, but the vast majority of people don't have this issue and can benefit greatly from the rich and easy offerings of dairy.

2. No alcohol

Alcohol is not exactly the devil, but it also is not the healthiest thing in the world. If you are trying to eat clean, you don't want to add any more stress to your liver than necessary, especially since it's already doing a Herculean job of scrubbing your blood of toxins. Yes, red wine can be healthy with its dose of the antioxidant resveratrol, but drinking too much of it and other types of alcohol can burden your body and impede it from carrying out many more important functions. But if you're still looking for that resveratrol, you have options. You can find it in grapes, peanuts, blueberries, cranberries, and pistachios.

3. No soda

This is the biggest NO on the plan. Despite the taste that many enjoy, soda has *absolutely* no redeeming qualities at all. Full of sugar, artificial sweeteners, additives, and other mystery chemicals, it is like drinking fizzy poison. If soda is something you regularly drink, just cutting it out will make you feel like a new person. I have had hundreds if not thousands of people either write to me or tell me in person how cutting soda from their diet completely turned things around for them. If you really need the carbonation, try some fizzy water and squeeze in fresh citrus juice. It's not perfect, but it can help.

4. Only freshly squeezed juice

There is such a thing called natural sugar. Sugar that is found in freshly squeezed juice comes just as nature created it. Yes, it's still sugar, and yes, it still has calories, but it's what comes with the sugar that makes the difference. It's what I call the "sugar package." Vitamins and minerals and other phytonutrients come along with the sugar in fresh juice and are paramount at boosting our health. If you're going to consume sugar, at least get some nutritional bang for your buck. One tip is, if it's possible, get freshly squeezed juice that hasn't been completely strained of the pulp and fruit skin, which contain lots of nutrients. Be careful of the labeling. For the purposes of the Clean 20, you should not be drinking anything from concentrate or major manufacturer brands that just say "100% juice." You should be looking for juices that are "freshly squeezed" and are labeled "no sugar added." The ingredients should only list juice from fruit or fruits and in some cases water, but nothing else.

5. Unlimited water

Water is one of the most magical natural health wonders on earth. It comprises up to 70% of our body, and while it doesn't contain the nutrients you find in food, it is essential for our very existence. It has no calories, helps energize muscles, keeps our skin looking good, helps our kidneys eliminate wastes, and gives a helping hand in maintaining normal bowel function. Most people don't drink enough water, but for the next twenty days you're going to find out what it feels like to really hydrate your body all the way down to the cells. Just because you drink to quench your thirst it doesn't mean you're drinking enough. For the next twenty days you should be consuming between 8 and 10 cups per day. No water with artificial sweeteners or added chemicals. If you want sparkling water, that's completely fine. If you want to squeeze some fresh citrus in your water, that's fine also. Keep it natural and abundant and your body will be grateful.

6. No added sugar

While sugar is often vilified, and for good reason, it still plays an important role in our body. Glucose (sugar) is actually the number one source of energy for our brain. Glucose is important energy for our muscles and the billion cellular processes that take place in our bodies every second of the day. But we are consuming an extraordinarily dangerous amount that is taking a toll on our health. Added sugar is the biggest culprit—it's the sugar you add to your foods at the table or that manufacturers slip into the foods while cooking or processing them. For the next twenty days, we are going to free our bodies of all this extra sugar, and you will notice the difference in your energy levels, complexion, and mood. The first few days might be challenging, but your body is an extremely adaptable machine and it will reconfigure so that, in short order, you will no longer crave that sweet stuff.

7. No artificial sweeteners

This should go without saying, but sometimes the most obvious things still need to be said. "Artificial" is a forbidden word for the next twenty days. While these sweeteners don't have any calories, that's the end of their good attributes. Scientists have raised all kinds of concerns, from them increasing your risk for something called the metabolic syndrome to increasing your affinity or addiction to even sweeter foods. Avoid them at all costs and make sure you read the labels carefully, as manufacturers can be very tricky when including them on the labels for their products, making them difficult to identify.

8. Fruits and vegetables are your friends

You might find yourself in a situation where you can't find a food on your list because it's simply not available. Not a problem. You are allowed to eat any fruit or vegetable even if they're not on your list. You can eat them raw or cooked, but if they are going to be cooked, make sure that they are not cooked in anything but olive oil with some spices. You can add as wide a variety of fruits and vegetables as you like, even if it pushes your list beyond twenty. These power foods are the absolute essence of clean eating!

9. No MSG

Monosodium glutamate is the salt version of the amino acid glutamate. While MSG can occur naturally in foods such as tomatoes and cheeses, it's often synthesized in the laboratory for commercial reasons. This synthetic MSG is used around the world as a flavor enhancer, commonly added to canned vegetables, soups, processed meats, and Chinese food. While the FDA has classified it as a food ingredient that's "generally regarded as safe," it remains at the center of many a food controversy. There have been many anecdotal reports of reactions to MSG, including headaches, heart palpitations (rapid, fluttering heartbeat), nausea, chest pain, weakness, and sweating. If these reactions are actually due to the MSG, they have been mild and short-lived. The FDA requires that foods containing MSG list it in the ingredients label on the packaging as "monosodium glutamate."

10. No frying

We don't want to take nature's clean, health-promoting food and ruin all of the whole goodness that it brings. Deep-frying foods does just that and is counter to our mission. Yes, fried food tastes better to some, but so do well-seasoned grilled, baked, and sautéed foods. When food is fried, more calories are added to it, because the food absorbs the fat of the cooking oils. It's okay to use olive oil to cook your food, as it is quite healthy and can enhance the nutritional value of your dish. However, cooking means sautéing your food or any preparation that is quick and doesn't subject or saturate the food to sustained high heat for a long period of time—that is the equivalent of frying.

11. No white flour

Flour is a perfect example of taking something completely nutritious and health-promoting and destroying it. The whole-wheat grain kernel is typically milled or processed (refined) and broken down into tiny pieces. In most instances, the process completely separates the three main parts of the kernel (bran, germ, endosperm). In the case of white flour, the endosperm is the only part of the three that is used, while the other two are thrown away. This basically means that the body will treat white flour as a starch and it will have similar effects in the body as eating refined sugar. Whole-wheat flour recombines the germ and bran with the endosperm further along in the process. While whole-wheat flour is absolutely more nutritious, it still has undergone refinement. It would be really difficult to live the rest of your life without consuming flour, since it's so prevalent in our foods, but for the next twenty days we are going to do our best to reduce our consumption as much as possible without it and give our overworked guts a little respite.

12. Careful with condiments

Ketchup, mustard, mayonnaise, and salsa are allowed, but there's a catch—the ketchup, mayonnaise, and salsa have to be home-made, so as to avoid mistakenly eating something that has been heavily processed. (See recipes, pages 232, 233, and 236) May-onnaise will not keep for the entire twenty days—it will last up to a week—so you will have to make it a couple of times. Mustard is more difficult to make without using processed ingredients and the finished product can taste quite different from the mustards you're accustomed to, so there is an allowance to purchase it. You can find several brands that make an organic product that doesn't use sugar or anything artificial. Just look at the back of the label and read the ingredients to make sure the brand fits the Clean 20 guidelines.

13. Canned and frozen are permitted

These items are allowed, but they must be clean. Nothing artifi-cial is allowed and they must be packaged in water or their natu-ral juices. Something like canned tuna in water is completely fine, as are organic frozen vegetables and fruits. With anything canned or frozen, always be mindful of the sodium content, as they tend to be high, so opt for low-sodium options. Before turning your nose up at frozen produce, you should be aware that the fresh fruit and vegetables you purchase at the store might not be as fresh as they look. In fact, a lot of produce is kept in storage for weeks at a time before it's put out for retail. Some fruits and veggies can lose up to 75% of a certain nutrient after sitting in storage for a week or more, because while they may look fresh externally, there's internal degradation occurring the whole time thanks to enzymes that continue to work even after the fruit or vegetable is harvested. If you're in the market for frozen produce, search for products that have been "flash frozen." This means they have been frozen very quickly after being harvested, thus preserving the field-fresh taste and ensuring peak ripeness as well as the greatest nutrient density (more nutrients for fewer calories).

14. Salad dressings allowed with restrictions

It is better to make your own salad dressing for these twenty days, something that is not very difficult to do. If, however, you must purchase dressing, it should only be organic, with no sugar added, and no artificial ingredients. Make sure the dressing is either fat-free or low-fat, but read the label, as manufacturers tend to sneak a lot of sugar into these dressings. The best bet is to make your own dressing, which will take few ingredients and not much time. Try the simple recipes on pages 234 and 235 and you won't have to worry about not finding the correct dressing at the grocery store.

four

How the Clean 20 Works

This program is meant to be exciting, adventurous, purifying, and convenient. There are twenty principal ingredients that you will be consuming for twenty days, and there are plenty of snack combinations that you can choose from as you journey to better health. The Clean 20 is all about simplicity. Stick to these ingredients and they will deliver a tremendous amount of energy, greater nutrient density (lots of nutrition for fewer calories), and better fuel for your body's optimal performance.

The ingredients chosen for the plan have been carefully selected to deliver maximum results. Whether you're a vegan, vegetarian, carnivore, gluten-free, or anything else, you can find enough choices to satisfy you. Try to avoid making substitutions to your list unless you *absolutely* need to do so. If you want to increase your Clean 20 list by adding more items, feel free to do so as long as they meet the guidelines of the program. Remember, this is only a twenty-day program, so don't look at it as something restricting or frustrating. Be creative and open your mind to new tastes and ingredients and their combinations. In fact, you might try tasting various foods and ingredients on their own so that you can experience the raw flavor and appreciate how various textures and flavors come together to create the final product. This will open your palate and introduce a variety of ingredients such as spices, herbs, and specialty foods (such as spelt, bulgur, and quinoa) that you might never have tried before but now know that you enjoy. If you approach these twenty days with a positive frame of mind and look at the program as an opportunity rather than a penalty for previous poor lifestyle choices and behaviors, then you will fly through the program with pleasure and alacrity.

Daily Meal Plan

Each day a meal plan is set up for you to follow. The key to these meal plans is that you get to create the menus that work best for you. This is an important part of the plan's flexibility. Each day there will be suggested meal options: choose from those suggestions or make your own from the twenty ingredients. What is important, however, is that you pay attention to portion sizes. Part of eating cleaner is appropriate consumption. Crowding your plate, going back for seconds, eating until you can barely get up from the table—these are behaviors that set you back rather than propel you forward.

To increase diversity in your consumption, it's important not to eat the same meal or combination twice in one day. You might have an ingredient or two that you eat more than once, but if that's the case, make sure you eat them in recipes or combinations that are different from what you ate previously. Nothing bad is going to happen to you if you are repetitive with your choices, but remember that eating should be fun and exploration and experimentation is part of the process of discovering new ways to satisfy your palate. Through the course of each five days, your goal should be to have consumed all twenty ingredients at least once. Keep track of what you're eating by making hash marks next to the ingredient on your master Clean 20 list. Remember, these ingredients were specially selected for the health and taste benefits that they deliver.

Look over the whole plan before you begin. This will give you a sense of what to expect and how best to prepare. There are lots of options and decisions you will make. The general guideline is to choose the best combination of taste, nutritional value, and calorie level. This is not a diet plan in the classic sense of "restricted calories," but it is a plan that is mindful of calorie consumption, making sure that you are eating only as much as you need and not eating to the point of overindulgence.

Breakfast

This is the most important meal of the day, despite the fact that so many people skip it. It's like fueling up your car and checking the oil levels before setting out on a long journey. Breakfast literally sets you up for the rest of the day, so taking the time to consider what you're having and actually eating it is extremely important. You are not required to eat all of the food that is listed, but you should eat at least some of it. If you're not a breakfast person, you might opt for the lighter fare such as smoothies or yogurt parfaits.

Lunch

There is no hard and fast time for lunch, but I suggest that you eat it no more than three hours after eating your breakfast. The lunch items are all interchangeable. If you see a lunch item from day 5 that you like and you are only on day 2, you're more than welcome to make the change.

Dinner

Try to think about dinner in advance. If you're going out to eat, think about where you're going and whether you'll be able to find the foods that you need. If not, then try to either eat something before you go or, if you have limited options, simply choose a clean salad. You don't have to eat a heavy dinner, as it is your last meal of the day—since it's not likely you will be able to burn it off, make sure you're eating until satisfied, not stuffed.

Beverages

The Clean 20 is all about fueling your body properly and eliminating additives and processed ingredients. Beverages are a big weakness for many people, because they often think that eating better only means improving the foods they consume. It's also about what you drink, as liquids are a prime source of hidden dangers. Added sugars, high calories, chemical concoctions, artificial ingredients—almost all commercially prepared beverages are loaded with substances that harm us in small ways, and that over time can deliver serious health consequences.

So, for these twenty days we are going to treat beverages just as we would treat the fuel we'd put into our car's gas tank. For our car to work best and for the engine and other parts to have the greatest chance of operating at peak performance and lasting as long as possible, we buy expensive fuel that is specifically designed for those goals to be met. The same is true of the gas we put in our bodies. Water is key to our existence. While it doesn't contain nutrients as fruits and vegetables do, we can't live without it, and not drinking enough of it can cause serious health problems. Feel free to drink as much of it as you want each day (unless your doctor is restricting your intake for medical reasons such as congestive heart failure or end stage kidney disease), but definitely try to consume at least 6 cups per day. You can add sliced fruit or squeeze the juice from fresh fruit into it. You can have mineral water or seltzer water. Try to drink your water as clean as possible.

Alcohol, while not toxic in small doses, is banished on the Clean 20. We are going to give our overworked livers a break and a chance to focus on responsibilities other than metabolizing the liquor that we put into our system.

Snacks

The snacks in the daily meal plans are only suggestions. If you want to choose something from the snacks chapter (page 237), that's completely fine. If you want to choose something that's not in the book at all, please make sure it's a clean snack and follows the guidelines. Snacks are major pitfalls, so think carefully and stay focused.

Meal Timing

There is no hard and fast rule with regards to when you eat your meals. In general, you should try to eat breakfast within 90 minutes of getting up and a snack in between breakfast and lunch. You should not eat dinner within 90 minutes of going to sleep. You have a snack option if you get a little hungry after dinner, but make sure you keep that snack light, at around 100 calories or fewer. A little hunger is not bad and shouldn't always trigger a meal or eating. Water is your friend, so drink plenty of it to help you get through the mild hunger, and if that doesn't do the trick, go ahead and grab a light snack.

Substitutions

If you have an allergy or simply can't find a certain food item, by all means make substitutions, but be smart about it. Don't substitute unhealthy foods outside of the guidelines if you need to make a swap. You can eat any of the meals at any time of the day, so if you want dinner for lunch and lunch for breakfast, that's up to you and acceptable. You can even look at days in the future and substitute for those meals. The Clean 20 is flexible to accommodate a variety of lifestyles and situations, so you can thoroughly enjoy eating and meal planning.

■ ■ ■ ■ ■ ■ ■ ■ ■ ■ ■ ■ ■ ■ ■

five

The Clean 20
Daily Meal Plan

This meal plan is based on my suggested Clean 20 list. *Your* actual meal plan might look different if you choose different ingredients for your list. Remember, you can add to your list as much as you want as long as those new items meet the guidelines set up in the Clean 20 Rules, beginning on page 77. Use the meal plan below as a template and make your own enough in advance so that you know what ingredients you need to purchase and which recipes you might try. For example, where I might have collard greens and zucchini as the vegetables for a certain meal, you might instead want carrots and squash. It is completely fine to choose your own items and just use mine as a guide. This will not change the effectiveness of the plan. One of the biggest keys to success is planning, so take the time to get yourself oriented and prepared, then execute the plan.

DAY 1: RESET

Hitting the reset button is an extremely powerful experience. All the lessons you have learned from your mistakes and things you've wished you had done differently can suddenly become your reality. Imagine a painter locked in an empty room with no art supplies. Despite his inability to express his artistic vision, his imagination remains robust and he still creates in his mind what he can't put on canvas. Finally, he is released from the room and returns to his painter's studio, where he is free to paint all of those creations bursting in his mind. For the next twenty days, *you* are that painter with an opportunity to express and conduct yourself in ways that until now might've only existed in your head. Past failures and shortcomings are only relevant now because they give context. Maintain a positive attitude and the confidence that if you can do it, great things will happen. Some things in life don't allow a second chance, but this is not one of them. Take a deep breath, collect yourself, and get ready to transform in ways that you never thought possible. This is your journey—go for it with great energy and boundless optimism!

Breakfast

Choose one of the following:

- 2 scrambled eggs with ⅓ cup diced veggies cooked with extra-virgin olive oil
- Omelet made with 2 eggs with ¼ cup diced veggies

Side (choose one of the following):

- 1 slice 100% whole-wheat or 100% whole-grain toast
- ½ cup berries

Snack

Choose one of the following:

- Sliced cucumbers with hummus dip (or choose from Snack List, pages 237–240)
- 150 calories or less snack option

Lunch

- Grilled chicken sandwich on 100% whole-grain or 100% whole-wheat bread with lettuce, tomato, and Clean Mayonnaise (see recipe, page 233) or organic mustard
- Kale or spinach salad with tomatoes, quinoa, cucumbers, and beans

Snack

Choose one of the following:

- Sliced tomatoes with pinch of pepper and/or salt and extra-virgin olive oil
- 150 calories or less snack option

Dinner

Choose one of the following:

- 1 cup whole-wheat spaghetti with squash or zucchini slices (3 ounces diced chicken or fish optional)
- 6 ounces grilled or baked fish with ½ cup roasted brussels sprouts and ½ cup steamed carrots

Snack (if desired)

- 100 calories or less snack option

Let's Get Physical

- 15,000 steps

- 5 flights of steps (A trip up and down is considered to be one flight; each flight should have 10 steps or more. See page 244.)
- 150 jumping jacks (If you have knee problems or can't do a full jumping jack, do a modified jumping jack where you don't have to jump off the ground but rather step to the side instead. You don't have to do all of the jumping jacks at once. You can break them up into smaller groups—like 15 or 30—and keep doing the smaller groups until you complete 150.)

FOOD FOR THOUGHT

Spirited Spinach

Beyond its great flavor and versatility, spinach is loaded with nutrients such as niacin, zinc, protein, fiber, iron, and vitamins A, C, E, and K. But it also contains folate, a B-vitamin (B9) that's naturally present in many foods, but also is available as a dietary supplement in a different form called folic acid. Our body critically needs folate, especially to make DNA and other genetic material and for the body's cells to divide. The Institute of Medicine recommends consuming 400 mcg daily. What happens when you don't get enough? Folate deficiency may lead to the development of major depression, and if you're taking antidepressant medications, it may cause reduced absorption and poor response to treatment. One cup of cooked spinach supplies you with more than half (263 mcg) of your daily value.

DAY 2: EXPECT

One of the easiest ways to ruin the satisfying experience of progress is to have unrealistic expectations. Expectations are at the core of motivation. It's normal and completely acceptable to undertake a task and have expectations about the results. But it starts to get unproductive when expectations are out of alignment with the practical. If a nine-year-old boy diligently practiced his basketball dribbling five days a week for a year, then said to his parents, "I expect to be a professional basketball player by the time I'm sixteen," it would be fair to say he had a quite unrealistic expectation. It's great that he wants to practice and hone his skills so that he will be a better player and achieve success, but it's not so great that his marker for success is so unattainable. So, after all of his hard work over this seven-year period, if he isn't drafted by a professional basketball team in high school, does that ruin how he can appreciate the great progress he has made? It's great to have dreams, but you must also have a healthy dose of realism so that you can still appreciate what you've accomplished even if you fall short of your dream. Expectations over these next twenty days can be a motivating force to keep you going and urge you toward making good decisions. But be realistic about where you're going to land, and be extremely grateful for every small victory along the way.

Breakfast

Choose one of the following:

- Avocado toast made with 2 slices sprouted-grain or 100% whole-wheat bread with ¼ avocado, mashed

- 8 ounces low-fat or fat-free organic Greek yogurt with ½ cup sliced strawberries (or other berries), 1 tablespoon chopped walnuts

Side (choose one of the following):

- 1 piece of whole fruit
- ½ cup berries

Snack

- ½ cucumber (about 8 slices) and hummus, or 150 calories or less snack option

Lunch

Choose one of the following:

- Tuna salad sandwich on 100% whole-wheat bread (mix ½ can tuna, 1 teaspoon Clean Mayonnaise (see recipe, page 233), 1 teaspoon low-fat or fat-free organic Greek yogurt, diced celery, diced sweet pickle) with 1 serving vegetables
- 1½ cups lentil, tomato, cucumber, or chicken soup with 1 serving vegetables

Snack

Choose one of the following:

- ½ cup raw or cooked veggies
- 150 calories or less snack option

Dinner

Choose one of the following:

- 5 ounces grilled skinless chicken breast with spinach and carrots

- Vegetarian plate with 3 servings vegetables (chickpeas, squash, spinach, broccoli) and 1 cup cooked quinoa

Snack (if desired)

- 100 calories or less snack option

Let's Get Physical

- 12,000 steps
- 4 flights of steps (A trip up and down is considered to be one flight; each flight should have 10 steps or more. See page 246.)
- 100 jumping jacks (If you have knee problems or can't do a full jumping jack, do a modified jumping jack where you don't have to jump off the ground but rather step to the side instead.)
- 3 sets of 10 squats (see page 246)

FOOD FOR THOUGHT

Bravo Broccoli

Calcium is linked to strong bones and strong teeth. The Institute of Medicine recommends that people aged nineteen to seventy-one years old consume 1000 mg per day and those over 71 years old consume 1200 mg on a daily basis. Most people automatically think of milk when searching for high-calcium foods, but don't underestimate the power of broccoli. It contains almost as much calcium as whole milk and, in fact, studies have found that the calcium in broccoli as well as some other dark leafy green vegetables is better absorbed by the body than the calcium found in milk. You hear the mention of vitamin C and you immediately think of your mother telling you to drink your orange juice. But oranges—for all the attention they get—have nothing on broccoli when it comes to vitamin C. Those green little trees contain as much as twice the amount of vitamin C as an orange.

DAY 3: BELIEVE

Very little is possible in life without belief. Whether it's believing you can successfully plant a garden, lower your golf handicap, or run a mile in less than nine minutes, belief is the intangible "X" factor for success. There are times when you can take two people with equal preparation, equal skillsets, equal desire, and equal opportunity, yet one succeeds and the other doesn't. There can be many reasons why the results vary between the two, but often it comes down to how much a person believes in himself or herself. It's critical over these next twenty days that you harbor this belief. When doubts seep in or obstacles stand in your way, belief is going to keep you from giving up. There is a certain amount of trust that is imperative when you try a new plan for the first time. Even with the best intentions and the finest plan, there's a lot that can go wrong or derail your efforts. This is why faith—and yes, sometimes it's a blind faith—is such an important ingredient to have in the mix. You might not see the results as fast as you want or in the way that you expect them to appear, but you must keep believing that if you execute the plan good things will happen. Sometimes all we have is belief, and in the most trying of times when the odds seem stacked against you, trust that the process will deliver and keep you on the path to success.

Breakfast

Choose one of the following:

- Berry Delight Smoothie (see recipe, page 174)
- Egg white omelet made from 2 eggs with ¼ cup diced veggies

Side (choose one of the following):

- 100% whole-wheat or 100% whole-grain English muffin
- 1 piece of fruit

Snack

Choose one of the following:

- 1 nonfat mozzarella cheese stick with a small apple
- 150 calories or less snack option

Lunch

Choose one of the following:

- Baja salad (mixture of 4-ounce grilled skinless chicken breast, chopped; 1 medium tomato, diced; ¼ cup black beans; ½ avocado, diced; 1 tablespoon chopped red onion; 1 teaspoon cilantro leaves; 1 tablespoon extra-virgin olive oil; juice of 1 lime)
- Large green garden salad sprinkled with ¼ cup chopped walnuts and shredded carrots

Snack

Choose one of the following:

- ⅓ cup wasabi peas
- 150 calories or less snack option

Dinner

Choose one of the following:

- 5 ounces grilled salmon with ½ cup squash and ½ cup quinoa
- 1 cup whole-wheat pasta with cooked vegetables and 3 ounces diced chicken

Snack (if desired)

- 100 calories or less snack option

Let's Get Physical

REST DAY (Still try to complete 8,000 steps or more.)

■ ■

FOOD FOR THOUGHT
Eggs

■ ■

The average American consumes more than 250 eggs over the course of the year, and for good reason. Eggs not only are tasty to many, but they contain the highest quality food protein known, second only to mother's milk for human nutrition. There are other foods that have more protein, but not the same quality. All parts of an egg are edible, including the shell, which has a high calcium content. Many people wash their eggs, but according to the USDA, it's not necessary because of the increased risk of introducing microbes (germs) into the egg through the pores of the shell. As the hen is laying her eggs, she coats them in a protective coating called a "bloom." The bloom seals the egg, keeping the germs out and the moisture in. When you crack the egg and the white part (albumin) appears cloudy, don't worry. This indicates the egg is very fresh. In fact, as time goes on the albumin becomes less cloudy and actually starts to clear. Egg yolks range in color from pale to deep orange. The color changes based on the hen's diet. Eggs that are fed plants eat more carotenoids—natural pigments like beta-carotene. The important thing to remember is that the macronutrients protein and fat remain the same regardless of the yolk color.

DAY 4: PREPARE

If the execution stage of a plan is the most critical part of its success, then the preparation phase is an extremely close second. Whether it's about taking a test, going on a long trip, or following a new eating plan, how well you prepare for the imminent task will have a direct and substantial impact on the outcome. My high school basketball coach had an adage that he would often repeat to us during practice. He called it the five Ps: Proper Preparation Prevents Poor Performance. He instilled in us the understanding that how we practiced was how we were ultimately going to play when it counted in a real game. So, while it was okay to have fun as we went through the drills, it was also important to stay focused and think about the situations we would encounter in a game and practice how we would handle them. These five Ps are critical to your success over the almost three weeks of the Clean 20. If you wait until the last minute to see what it is you need to eat or what exercises you need to do, then there's a tremendously high likelihood that you will not follow the plan tightly or fit in all you need to do for that day. One of the biggest pitfalls for people embarking on a new eating regime is that they don't properly think ahead and find themselves in an environment that is not conducive to their new eating strategy. There's a saying that "an ounce of prevention is worth a pound of cure." Well, "ten minutes of planning prevents an hour of stress." You will find the most success and the most comfort when you take those precious few minutes to think about what's ahead of you and what you need to do to stay on track.

Breakfast

Choose one of the following:

- 1 cup oatmeal with blueberries and 1 teaspoon honey
- 1 bowl of mixed fruit (diced apples, pineapples, melon, and oranges)

Side (choose one of the following):

- 6 ounces low-fat or fat-free organic Greek yogurt
- 1 piece of fruit
- 1 slice 100% whole-grain or 100% whole-wheat toast

Snack

Choose one of the following:

- 1 apple or 1 orange
- 150 calories or less snack option

Lunch

Choose one of the following:

- Avocado sandwich with 2 slices 100% whole-grain bread; ¼ avocado, mashed; 1 ounce cheese; 2 tomato slices
- 5-ounce veggie burger on 100% whole-grain bun with lettuce, tomato, and onion and small green garden salad

Snack

Choose one of the following:

- 1 carrot, sliced (or 6 baby carrots), with 2 tablespoons hummus
- 150 calories or less snack option

Dinner

Choose one of the following:

- Whole-wheat rigatoni pasta with Turkey Meatballs (see recipe, page 205)
- 5 ounces grilled or baked cod with ½ cup cauliflower and ½ cup green beans

Snack (if desired)

- 100 calories or less snack option

Let's Get Physical

- 14,000 steps
- 7 flights of steps (A trip up and down is considered to be one flight; each flight should have 10 steps or more. See page 246.)
- 3 minutes of jog punches (see page 248)
- 3 minutes of ice skaters (see page 243)

DAY 5: FOCUS

It's very easy to make a plan, get excited about following the plan, get everything ready to maximize your chance for success, then get distracted and not make good on your intentions. Being able to stay focused is definitely not as easy as it might sound, but it's imperative if you're going to fend off those temptations that can divert you from the path of success. Every morning before starting your day, you should take three to five minutes and review in your mind the day's flow of activities and what you need to do to make it as smooth and productive as possible. Remind yourself of your reasons for deciding to make this life change and recommit yourself to doing what it takes to succeed. I was watching a tennis match at the 2017 US Open between the world number-one player Rafael Nadal and a player ranked eighty-five, Dušan Lajović. The beginning of the match was mesmerizing as Lajović took it hard to Nadal and never flinched. Aggressive, fearless, and full of adrenaline, he was hitting amazing shots and winning in front of a stunned crowd. Then as the match wore on, things changed—slowly at first, but then in a rapid transformation. Lajović was no longer making those amazing shots and Nadal was finally getting into the groove. It was a spectacular dichotomy of focus on both sides of the net—a sudden reversal, where focus was disastrously lost by Lajović and impressively gained by Nadal. Once Nadal took the lead, he never looked back and easily claimed victory. This is an instructive tale for anyone trying to execute a game plan. Unlike Lajović, who had focus only in the beginning of the match when his adrenaline was charging him along, you must keep your focus throughout the twenty days when the initial excitement and novelty of your mission have worn off. The force of your conviction will power you to the end.

Breakfast

Choose one of the following:

- Baked Apple Oatmeal Cups (see recipe, page 177)
- 2 slices 100% whole-grain toast with organic nut butter and sliced apples

Side (choose one of the following):

- 2 strips turkey bacon
- 1 piece of fruit

Snack

Choose one of the following:

- ¼ cup walnuts (or peanuts, cashews, almonds, or pecans)
- 150 calorie or less snack option

Lunch

Choose one of the following:

- 1½ cups tomato or cucumber or black bean soup with small green garden salad
- Herb-encrusted grilled skinless chicken breast with salad greens

Snack

Choose one of the following:

- 8 black olives
- 150 calories or less snack option

Dinner

Choose one of the following:

- Herb-Encrusted Grilled Tuna Steak (see recipe, page 217)
- Whole-wheat spaghetti and Turkey Meatballs (see recipe, page 205)

Snack (if desired)

- 100 calories or less snack option

Let's Get Physical

- 17,000 steps
- 150 jumping jacks (If you have knee problems or can't do a full jumping jack, do a modified jumping jack where you don't have to jump off the ground but rather step to the side instead.)
- 3 minutes of high knees (see page 244)
- 3 minutes of ice skaters (see page 243)
- 3 sets of 10 squats (see page 246)

■ ■

FOOD FOR THOUGHT

Cheaper Than You Think

■ ■

Most people believe that produce, while extremely healthy, can also be extremely expensive. In fact, many use this as a reason for buying more processed packaged foods. Well, not so fast. The U.S. Department of Agriculture found that a serving of cookies and crackers costs about 30 cents, but a serving of produce costs approximately 25 cents. Not only are fruits and vegetables cheaper than some of the less-healthy fare, but they are high in fiber and fill you up longer so you're not always reaching for something else to eat.

DAY 6: CLEANSE

These twenty days will be about cleansing your body and environment of foods, drinks, situations, and even people who are preventing you from becoming the best you. There are some environmental factors in our daily lives that we can't control—weather, your boss, the late arrival of the commuter train. But there are other things that are firmly within grasp and under your control that you can regulate immediately. The first things to get rid of are conditions that are temptations. Go to your cabinet and throw or give away all of the foods that are not part of your next twenty days. You might be inclined to leave it there with a promise to yourself that you won't touch them. For the extremely disciplined and focused, this might work, but for the vast majority of people, the knowledge that these foods are readily available becomes an overwhelming distraction, to the point that it seduces them at their weakest moment. Second, there are constant reminders in our lives that make us feel a range of emotions. For these twenty days, you want to spend your energy in creating and living in a positive space. Lastly, there might be people or objects that are going to drag you into negativity. If you can't completely remove them from your life, at least reduce the amount of your contact time. You want to remove as many obstacles as possible so that your highway to happiness and success is unobstructed!

Breakfast

Choose one of the following:

- 1 cup grits with 1 ounce cheese (optional)
- Grilled cheese sandwich on 100% whole-grain bread and 2 to 3 ounces cheese

Side (choose one of the following):

- 1 piece of fruit
- 6 ounces low-fat or fat-free organic Greek yogurt

Snack

Choose one of the following:

- 20 raw almonds
- 150 calories or less snack option

Lunch

Choose one of the following:

- 5-ounce turkey burger with lettuce and tomato on 100% whole-grain bun
- Large green garden salad with 2 tablespoons clean dressing (see recipes, pages 234 and 235)

Snack

Choose one of the following:

- 2 tablespoons pumpkin or sesame seeds
- 150 calories or less snack option

Dinner

Choose one of the following:

- Seared Herbed Sea Bass (see recipe, page 214)
- Vegetable or turkey meat lasagna ($4 \times 2 \times 1\frac{1}{2}$ inches)

Snack (if desired)

- 100 calories or less snack option

Let's Get Physical

- REST DAY (Still try to complete 8,000 steps or more.)

FOOD FOR THOUGHT

Nut Power

According to the Global Burden of Disease Study, which involved nearly 500 researchers and 100,000 data sources, not eating enough nuts and seeds kills more people than processed meat consumption, and potentially leads to the deaths of fifteen times more people than all those who die from over-dosing on crack cocaine, heroin, and all other illicit drugs combined. Eating more vegetables could save 1.5 million lives. The study made these calculations from a variety of research data gathered across fifty countries. Researchers speculate that the health-promoting nutrients of nuts and vegetables are the reason why more lives would be saved if they were added to the diet.

Source: NutritionFacts.org.

DAY 7: VISUALIZE

Sam Snead was one of the greatest golfers to ever play the game. Whether or not you're a golf fan, there's a technique he used that you can employ in your own life as you tackle various endeavors. The pre-shot ritual in golf is one of the most important parts of the swing, as it calms the golfer down and gets him prepared to execute a shot. When asked about his ritual, Snead would say that he'd paint a picture in the sky of the shot he planned to hit, then step up and try to mimic what he had just painted. Jack Nicklaus, another of the world's greatest golfers, said that before hitting the ball he would take a moment so that he would clearly see the shot shape, trajectory, and even how the ball would react when landing. This process of seeing the result before attempting to achieve it is something that you can effectively apply over this clean journey. Visualize what is happening externally and internally as you choose healthier options and commit yourself to a regular routine of physical activity. Think about how your skin will be better hydrated and blemishes disappearing, your liver not having to work overtime to clean your blood of so many chemicals and toxins, your muscles gaining strength and size, and your brain being flushed with powerful nutrients that will keep it healthy and agile. The foods and beverages you consume will have a direct impact on how you feel and function, so imagine all of those tiny cells throughout your body getting excited about the clean fuel they are receiving as you make smart choices. See what you want to happen and it will become your reality.

Breakfast

Choose one of the following:

- Heavenly Blueberry Oatmeal (see recipe, page 183)
- Tropical smoothie bowl (pulse banana, mango, pineapple, and almond milk until smooth and thick; top with blueberries, fresh kiwi, and peaches)

Side (choose one of the following):

- ½ cup sliced fruit
- 1 slice 100% whole-grain or 100% whole-wheat toast with organic preserves

Snack

Choose one of the following:

- 1 piece of fruit
- 150 calories or less snack option

Lunch

Choose one of the following:

- 1½ cups whole-wheat spaghetti with sun-dried tomatoes and 3 ounces grilled chicken strips
- 3 servings cooked vegetables

Snack

Choose one of the following:

- 1 hard-boiled egg sprinkled with salt and choice of spices (pepper, paprika, etc.)
- 150 calories or less snack option

Dinner

Choose one of the following:

- Spicy Grilled Chicken (see recipe, page 211)
- Large green garden salad with ½ cup black beans and 4 ounces fish cut into chunks (chicken or turkey strips can be substituted for the fish)

Snack (if desired)

- 100 calories or less snack option

Let's Get Physical

- 12,000 steps
- 7 flights of steps (A trip up and down is considered to be one flight; each flight should have 10 steps or more. See page 246.)
- 200 jumping jacks (If you have knee problems or can't do a full jumping jack, do a modified jumping jack where you don't have to jump off the ground but rather step to the side instead.)
- 3 minutes of planks (Don't try to do 3 minutes at once. Instead, do it in subsets such as 30 seconds at a time until you've completed the 3 minutes. See page 248.)

FOOD FOR THOUGHT

The Odd Couple (Iron & Vitamin C)

Like most things in life, more is accomplished by a team that works well together than the individual efforts of a lone superstar. Iron is needed to maintain a healthy immune system and energy levels. Iron is primarily found in meats, poultry, seafood, vegetables, and legumes. The body can easily absorb iron from meats, but not so easily from vegetables and legumes. This is where vitamin C steps in and does its job, breaking down the iron into parts so that the body has an easier time absorbing it. Some examples of these odd pairings are oatmeal and blueberries, lentils and red bell peppers, and dark leafy greens with lemon juice.

DAY 8: ENJOY

Sometimes it's easy to forget about the essence of life—joy. We get so bogged down in the process of "doing" that we forget about the state of "being" and how important it is to enjoy where we are and not always look to where we want to be. A joyless effort or result seems counter to what the mission should be. It's wonderful to reach a goal, but if the process is rife with displeasure or feels onerous, the victory is diminished. Finding those pockets of happiness can go a long way, as evidenced in many studies looking at the relationship between employee happiness and productivity. One study conducted by a team of economists at the University of Warwick in England found that employee happiness led to a 12% spike in productivity, while unhappy workers proved to be 10% less productive. While your work on the Clean 20 doesn't have the rigors of a job, there *are* challenges you will face. It's not easy to make dietary changes when you've been accustomed to eating or drinking a particular way for a long period of time. However, as you're trying to steer clear of potential land mines and pitfalls, it's important not to take things too seriously and to have fun. Sometimes a good laugh or a moment of shrugging your shoulders at a temporary setback can make all the difference in whether you continue to move forward in a positive manner or become permanently derailed. There will be circumstances and moments during this journey that will test you, but roll with it and keep finding ways to have fun. A positive attitude can help you weather the most severe of storms.

Breakfast

Choose one of the following:

- Scrambled eggs and tomato sandwich with a drizzle of extra-virgin olive oil (2 scrambled eggs and thinly sliced tomatoes on 100% whole-wheat bread)
- Breakfast Smoothie (350 calories or less; see recipes, pages 172 to 174)

Side (choose one of the following):

- 1 piece of fruit
- ½ cup berries

Snack

Choose one of the following:

- 3 cups air-popped popcorn
- 150 calories or less snack option

Lunch

Choose one of the following:

- 6-ounce piece of grilled or baked fish with ½ cup zucchini slices and ½ cup collard greens
- 1½ cups soup with small green garden salad

Snack

Choose one of the following:

- 6 ounces low-fat or fat-free organic Greek yogurt
- 150 calories or less snack option

Dinner

Choose one of the following:

- Lemon Pasta with Chicken (see recipe, page 226) or Pesto chicken and zucchini spaghetti
- Lasagna made with whole-wheat pasta with small green garden salad (if you can't find whole-wheat lasagna noodles, try buckwheat noodles, spelt pasta, quinoa pasta, or brown rice pasta)

Snack (if desired)

- 100 calories or less snack option

Let's Get Physical

- 16,000 steps
- 3 minutes of jog punches (see page 248)
- 3 minutes of high knees (see page 244)
- 3 minutes of running in place
- 3 minutes of steam engines (see page 247)

FOOD FOR THOUGHT

Triumphant Tomato Paste

Tomatoes are beloved around the world for their juicy rich flavor and the many varieties used in different cooking preparations. Their star nutrient is lycopene, a carotenoid that is a naturally occurring chemical that gives fruits and vegetables a red color. They're also considered to be an antioxidant (disease preventer and fighter) that protects cells from damage. Some studies have shown they can even help prevent prostate cancer. While tomato and tomato paste are both full of lycopene, typical reasoning would follow that the lycopene in the raw, natural tomato would be better than that found in tomato paste. Not so. In fact, research shows that the bioavailability (amount that gets absorbed in the body) of lycopene is greater from tomato paste than from fresh tomatoes.

DAY 9: BALANCE

Finding the right balance in your life can be tricky. Most of us have so many things we are trying to juggle that sometimes we feel suffocated by the pressure to get it all done and to get it done well. The first two things you need to accept is that joy must come before perfection and that sometimes having it all really can mean having less. As you embark on a journey to better health, you need to understand that making perfect decisions in what you eat and how you move is not a requirement and, in fact, could be a self-defeating goal. Try your best to remain true to your purpose, but remember that there's a lot more to life than what's on your plate or in your cup. There are going to be moments when you have to make a tough decision. Maybe you find yourself in a food environment with no good choices or have someone waiting for you and you know this will mean not having enough time to get your physical activity in for the day. This happens and this is life. There's no need to beat yourself up about it and stress about not being able to do it all. Remember to stop yourself from getting anxious. Play an instrument, read a book, listen to music, go for a walk—do anything that you enjoy and that will reduce your anxiety. Find that balance that keeps you moving forward, do the best you can, and keep it all in perspective.

Breakfast

Choose one of the following:

- Easy Egg Frittata (see recipe, page 176)
- Grilled cheese sandwich on 100% whole-grain bread with 2 to 3 ounces cheese

Side (choose one of the following):

- ½ cup melon slices
- 6 ounces low-fat or fat-free organic vanilla Greek yogurt with sliced fruit

Snack

Choose one of the following:

- 1 cup raw or cooked cauliflower with 2 tablespoons hummus
- 150 calories or less snack option

Lunch

Choose one of the following:

- Veggie or turkey burger with lettuce, tomato, and onion on 100% whole-grain bun with Homemade Ketchup or Clean Mayonnaise (see recipes, pages 232 and 233) and a small green garden salad
- Chicken sandwich on 100% whole-grain bread with tomato, lettuce, and 1 ounce cheese (optional) with Clean Mayonnaise (see recipe, page 233) or organic mustard
- 1½ cups vegetable juice and small green garden salad

Snack

Choose one of the following:

- ¾ cup steamed edamame
- 150 calories or less snack option

Dinner

Choose one of the following:

- Lemon-Drizzled Grilled Chicken (see recipe, page 210) with ½ cup bok choy and ½ cup red beans

- Vegetarian plate of 4 servings vegetables—pinto beans, cauliflower, spinach, and squash

Snack (if desired)

- 150 calories or less snack option

Let's Get Physical

- REST DAY (Still try to complete 8,000 steps or more.)

FOOD FOR THOUGHT

Breakfast Power

Nutritionists have argued for years that breakfast is the most important meal of the day. It is an important opportunity for the body to refuel and replenish after spending a considerable amount of time burning calories without taking in any nutrition. Although most U.S. consumers begin their day with breakfast, one out of ten, or 31 million, don't, according to a recent food market research study conducted by the NPD Group, a leading marketing research company. Males eighteen to thirty-four have the highest incidence of skipping (28%), whereas adults fifty-five and older have the lowest incidence of skipping among adults. Among children, the incidence of skipping increases as children age, with thirteen- to seventeen-year-olds having the highest incidence (14%) of skipping.

Source: NPD Group.

DAY 10: ORGANIZE

Just the word "organize" can create anxiety and trepidation. It conjures thoughts of effort and lots of time being consumed, with little to show for it. But the benefits of being organized are substantial. There is something exciting about spontaneity, the idea of doing whatever comes to mind and feeling free to make decisions as situations present themselves. However liberating this might feel, it can come at a cost. Your chances of success are diminished when you are not prepared for the unexpected. Over these twenty days, organizing your life will help you organize your meal and exercise plans, not only giving you a better shot at success, but making the process of accomplishing it feel less arduous. Here are three things you can try that can help deliver immediate benefits:

1. **Declutter.** Schedule a time either once a week or a couple of times a week to organize your physical things, whether it be your closet, basement storage room, or cabinets. Clearing out what you don't need or use can help clear out your mind and help you focus. And make sure everything has a proper home rather than the place it was just left because of convenience.

2. **Write it down.** In the fast-paced world of distractions and obligations we live in, committing everything we need to do to memory is not always a guarantee that we will recall what needs to be done at the right time. Write things down on old-fashioned paper or in the notes section of your smartphone. Besides helping you remember, the process of writing things down gives you another chance to think through whatever the task or goal is.

3. Be early. Remember, the best way to get something done is to begin. Too many times we procrastinate and wait till the last second to start or complete a task. Make a schedule, pay attention to the timing of the schedule, and rather than being on time or late, be early by five or ten minutes. There's no penalty for being ahead.

Breakfast

Choose one of the following:

- 2 scrambled eggs with 1 ounce cheese and 2 slices turkey bacon
- 1 cup oatmeal with 1 teaspoon honey

Side (choose one of the following):

- 1 apple, orange, or banana
- 1 slice 100% whole-grain toast
- ½ cup berries

Snack

Choose one of the following:

- 10 cherry tomatoes sprinkled with salt, pepper, and vinaigrette
- 150 calories or less snack option

Lunch

Choose one of the following:

- 6-ounce turkey burger with lettuce, tomato, onion, and cheese on a 100% whole-grain bun with 2 servings vegetables
- 1½ cups lentil, black bean, tomato, chicken, or vegetable soup with small green garden salad

Snack

Choose one of the following:

- 1 stick of celery, chopped, and 2 tablespoons hummus
- 150 calories or less snack option

Dinner

Choose one of the following:

- Grilled Chicken and Tomato-Lime Salsa (see recipe, page 212)
- Large green garden salad with 4 ounces chicken strips or sliced fish and 2 tablespoons clean salad dressing

Snack (if desired)

- 150 calories or less snack option

Let's Get Physical

- 15,000 steps
- 8 flights of steps (A trip up and down is considered to be one flight; each flight should have 10 steps or more. See page 246.)
- 3 minutes of running in place
- 3 minutes of steam engines (see page 247)

FOOD FOR THOUGHT
The Tea on Tea

Next to water, tea is the most widely consumed beverage in the world. In the U.S. alone, almost 80% of all households contain tea, and on any given day, over 158 million Americans are drinking this popular beverage. While green tea has been heralded in the media quite often, the most consumed variety is black tea, comprising almost 80% of all tea consumed. One of tea's unique qualities is that it is readily consumed either iced or hot, making it a convenient beverage for all types of occasions. What many might not know is that black, green, oolong, dark, and white teas all come from the same plant—*Camellia sinensis*—which is a warm-weather evergreen. Tea leaves go through a consistent process—plucked, laid out to dry or wither, rolled, oxidized, then "fired" or heated to stop the oxidation process. What makes each tea different is the amount of processing and level of oxidization. For example, black tea is considered to be "fully" oxidized while oolong tea is partially oxidized. Oxidation is a series of chemical reactions that occurs after the leaves are harvested and results in the browning of tea leaves and the production of aromatic compounds and flavor that can be found in finished teas. Manufacturers can control the oxidation process or prevent it altogether, as is the case with green and white tea leaves, which are not oxidized after their leaves are harvested. When it comes to strength and color, oolong tea is in between black and green.

Source: Tea Association of the USA, Inc.

DAY 11: PUSH

This marks the midway point of your twenty-day journey. This is quite a milestone to celebrate. Take a few minutes and look back at where you started and how far you've come. It's likely you had some doubts early in the process; you have probably thought at least a couple of times that it might be best to just throw in the towel and go back to eating and moving the way you have in the past. But your resilience and determination held you up, and look at how far you've come. One of the biggest mistakes people make during a journey is not looking back to see the ground they've covered. Perspective is never more important than when you need a springboard to help you launch even higher and farther. This midpoint is an opportunity to dig in even deeper, turn it up a notch, and push yourself to even greater heights. You've had ten days to get into a groove, so now you are very familiar with the plan and expectations. You should be settled into a nice comfortable routine. When you achieve a goal, it's easy to lose your edge and drive. Confidence can become a double-edged sword; it's important to believe that you can accomplish and succeed, but sometimes it can demotivate you and reduce your ambition to find new ways to win. Fight against this urge to fall back, and instead push yourself to make even better decisions by continuing to focus on making improvements so that there's a positive impact not only on this health journey, but on your life in general.

Breakfast

Choose one of the following:

- Egg and Turkey Casserole (see recipe, page 178)
- Smoothie or shake (350 calories or less)

Side (choose one of the following):

- 1 slice 100% whole-grain or 100% whole-wheat toast
- 6 ounces low-fat or fat-free plain organic Greek yogurt with fresh berries

Snack

Choose one of the following:

- 1 apple, sliced, with 1 tablespoon organic peanut butter
- 150 calories or less snack option

Lunch

Choose one of the following:

- 5 ounces grilled skinless chicken breast with ½ cup spinach and ½ cup cannellini beans
- 1½ cups turkey, tomato, lentil, bean, or cucumber soup

Snack

Choose one of the following:

- Egg salad sandwich: 1 whole egg, ½ teaspoon Clean Mayonnaise (page 233), and spices spread on slice of 100% whole-grain or 100% whole-wheat bread
- 150 calories or less snack option

Dinner

Choose one of the following:

- Sea Bass and Mango Salsa (see recipe, page 216)
- 12 oysters, ½ cup swiss chard, and ½ cup squash
- 1½ cups asparagus, bean, chickpea, chicken, or lentil soup

Snack (if desired)

- 100 calories or less snack option

Let's Get Physical

- REST DAY (Still try to complete 8,000 steps or more.)

FOOD FOR THOUGHT

Think Zinc

Zinc is an essential mineral shown to improve skin tone, help with wound healing, fight certain cancers, and shorten the length of time one suffers from the common cold. But zinc is also important for our brains. Researchers have identified the crucial role it plays in proper brain function and the prevention of cognitive decline as we age. The Institute of Medicine recommends consuming 11 milligrams per day for men nineteen years and older and 8 milligrams for women nineteen and over unless pregnant, in which case that number climbs to 11 milligrams. The best sources of this brain booster are beef, spinach, asparagus, mushrooms, oats, sesame seeds, pumpkin seeds, and seafood such as oysters and shrimp. Oysters contain more zinc per serving than any other food.

DAY 12: DECELERATE

Often when we have big expectations, the pressure causes us to race through the steps necessary to achieve the results we're seeking. This is why it's important sometimes to decelerate and slow things down. When you're watching an action sequence in a movie at home or a spectacular play in a sporting event, it's almost a reflex to grab the remote, rewind everything back to that important moment, then press the slow-motion button so that you can see and appreciate every frame with great clarity. That's what we need to do with life sometimes. There's so much going on with so many demands in such a short period of time that we don't get a chance to see and enjoy those precious frames. Take your time over these twenty days to slow down the process and truly appreciate the decisions you're making. Taste the ingredients of the food carefully and try to enjoy their different and unique flavors, then combine them in new, exciting ways. Take a moment to smile and savor even the smallest of personal victories you achieve along the way. One of my favorite sayings is "Life is not a sprint, but a marathon." This approach will help you enjoy the process of your transformation rather than see it as a chore.

Breakfast

Choose one of the following:

- Baked Oatmeal (see recipe, page 184)
- 2 slices 100% whole-grain or 100% whole-wheat toast spread with mashed avocado

Side (choose one of the following):

- 1 banana or pear, or ½ cup melon cubes
- 2 slices turkey bacon

Snack

Choose one of the following:

- 45 shelled pistachios
- 150 calories or less snack option

Lunch

Choose one of the following:

- Yummy Baked Tomatoes (see recipe, page 195) with 4 ounces fish or grilled skinless chicken
- Turkey sandwich on 100% whole-grain bread with 5 ounces turkey, with the option of 1 ounce cheese, tomato, lettuce, and organic mustard or Clean Mayonnaise (see recipe, page 233), and a side serving of raw or cooked vegetables

Snack

Choose one of the following:

- Watermelon skewers: take 6 toothpicks and on each place 1 cube watermelon, 1 small cube feta cheese, and 1 slice cucumber
- 150 calories or less snack option

Dinner

Choose one of the following:

- Proteinaceous Salmon Pasta (see recipe, page 227) with ½ cup spinach and ½ cup corn

- 4 servings cooked vegetables (corn, cabbage, black beans, and carrots) with ½ cup cooked quinoa

Snack (if desired)

- 100 calories or less snack option

Let's Get Physical

- 20,000 steps
- 3 minutes of steam engines (see page 247)
- 3 sets of 10 squats (see page 246)

FOOD FOR THOUGHT

Soda Sugar Bomb

Everyone knows that soda contains a lot of sugar, but many people don't know exactly *how* much. You can taste the sweetness, but you can't see it, and that prevents the drinker from having actual context. For example, let's take a 20-ounce bottle of Coca-Cola, a bottle size that many people consume very easily in one sitting. It contains 65 grams of sugar. Here's the context. When figuring out how many teaspoons of sugar are in a product, take the number of grams and divide by four. So in this case, 65 grams of sugar divided by four gives you 16.25 teaspoons of sugar. Think about lining up all those teaspoons of sugar and spooning them into your mouth the next time you consider reaching for that soda bottle.

DAY 13: MOVE

When most people think about changing their diet, they sometimes forget that diet's greatest companion is movement. While you focus on eating cleaner food and replenishing your cells with vital nutrients that make you feel better and ward off disease, don't discount the contribution that movement plays. A regular regimen of physical activity can affect almost every organ system in the body. It can help increase your muscle tone, improve your balance and stability, strengthen your muscles, reduce your risk of type 2 diabetes, reduce your risk for cardiovascular disease, help weight management, increase your chances of living longer, and improve your mood. In fact, exercise is a form of detoxification, as it increases the release of metabolic byproducts through the skin, through breathing, and by increasing the rate of blood flow through your vessels. Many people, unfortunately, think that going to the gym for an hour or more and working themselves into a state of utter exhaustion is the only way to make exercise worthwhile. While for some this might be beneficial, for many there are other options available that will deliver better results. Over these twenty days it's important that you also focus on your movement and the daily physical activity regimen that accompanies the meal plan. I've added suggestions for you, on each and every day of the plan (even on rest days), but if you want to do more, by all means go for it. The key is that whatever you decide to do, make sure you put forth a strong effort. Riding a stationary bike and reading a magazine at the same time is not the type of effort that will maximize results. Even if you only get physical for twenty minutes, give your all for every minute and the results will definitely come.

Breakfast

Choose one of the following:

- Energy Explosion Yogurt (see recipe, page 182)
- 1 cup mixed fruit with 3 tablespoons low-fat or fat-free organic vanilla Greek yogurt

Side (choose one of the following):

- ½ cup berries or 1 orange or 1 apple
- 1 slice 100% whole-grain or 100% whole-wheat toast

Snack

Choose one of the following:

- 7 olives stuffed with 1 tablespoon feta or blue cheese
- 150 calories or less snack option

Lunch

Choose one of the following:

- Succulent Turkey Burger (see recipe, page 200) with small green garden salad
- 1½ cups lentil, chickpea, tomato, or bean soup with small green garden salad

Snack

Choose one of the following:

- Cucumbers and hummus (slice ½ large cucumber and combine with 2 tablespoons hummus)
- 150 calories or less snack option

Dinner

Choose one of the following:

- Grilled Halibut with Tomatoes (see recipe, page 223)
- 6 ounces grilled fish or skinless chicken breast with ½ cup corn and ½ cup black beans

Snack (if desired)

- 100 calories or less

Let's Get Physical

- 12,000 steps
- 10 flights of steps (A trip up and down is considered to be one flight; each flight should have 10 steps or more. See page 246.)
- 3 minutes of planks (see page 248)
- 3 minutes of ice skaters (see page 243)

FOOD FOR THOUGHT

Copper Gold

It's difficult to imagine that the copper used for roof flashing and the wiring in your house is also important to health. Copper is a trace mineral—trace meaning that your body needs it in very small amounts. But copper is like gold when it comes to what it offers the body. It's found in every tissue of the body, but most of it is stored in the liver. Copper teams up with iron to help form red blood cells, but it also helps keep the immune system healthy, creates the coating for our nerve fibers, and assists in the development of melanin, the pigment that gives color to skin and hair. Most of us can get enough by eating a balanced diet. Some of the best sources include: crabs, oysters, squid, mussels, eggplants, mushrooms, dark leafy greens, sunflower seeds, cashews, and tofu.

DAY 14: RELAX

Go ahead and cue the song "Don't Worry, Be Happy": the sentiment and free-spirited rhythm of that soundtrack is a perfect
thread for our journey. It's okay to want to perform your best,
but it's also paramount that you reduce the pressure you place
on yourself. Perfectionism is a double-edged sword. It's a great
motivator to get you to give your best effort, but it's also a
stressor that can obscure the good that you'll accomplish even if
your ultimate goals aren't reached. Stress affects the respiratory
system, making breathing harder and raising levels of stress hormones that can increase heart rate and strengthen contractions of
heart muscles. Stress affects other physiological processes, including liver function, stomach sensations and function, digestion, the central nervous system, and the reproductive system.
This is why engaging a de-stressing activity on a daily basis is not
just good for your mind and mood, but important for full-body
relief. Start by taking just 30 minutes every day to allow your
mind and body to relax. It sounds like a small amount of time
given there are 24 hours available every day, but many people
have a difficult time finding even 15 minutes for themselves. For
30 minutes each day do something that directly and primarily
affects you and relaxes your mind, freeing it from the typical
stressors that come in the daily routine of life. Meditate in silence
or with soothing background music.

Breakfast

Choose one of the following:

- Nifty Bacon, Egg, and Cheese Sandwich (see recipe, page
  181)

- 2 scrambled eggs with extra-virgin olive oil with 1 ounce cheese and diced peppers or spinach

Side (choose one of the following):

- 2 slices turkey bacon
- 1 kiwi, ½ mango, or ½ cup berries

Snack

Choose one of the following:

- ¼ cup raw mixed nuts (unsalted)
- 150 calories or less snack option

Lunch

Choose one of the following:

- Tomato Chickpea Salad (see recipe, page 196)
- Tuna salad sandwich on 100% whole-grain or 100% whole-wheat bread with lettuce with ½ cup raw carrots and hummus

Snack

Choose one of the following:

- 20 seedless grapes with 10 almonds or cashews
- 150 calories or less snack option

Dinner

Choose one of the following:

- Whole-Wheat Spaghetti with Edamame Pesto Gusto (see recipe, page 187)

- 6 ounces grilled skinless chicken breast or turkey with ½ cup black-eyed peas and 6 to 8 roasted brussels sprouts

Snack (if desired)

- 100 calories or less snack option

Let's Get Physical

- REST DAY (Still try to complete 8,000 steps or more.)

FOOD FOR THOUGHT

Protein Punch

Turkey, fish, and cheese have the highest protein-to-calorie ratio. We know turkey and fish are packed with protein, but found it surprising that cheese contains just as much protein per calorie. For every 4.7 calories, you'll get 1 gram of protein. The cheeses with the most protein per calorie are low-fat mozzarella and cottage cheese. Here are some other foods with high protein to calorie ratios:

Lean turkey/chicken: 1 gram/4.6 calories
Lean beef: 1 gram/5.3 calories
Egg whites: 1 gram/4.7 calories
Tofu: 1 gram/7.4 calories
Hemp seeds: 1 gram/7.5 calories
Beans: 1 gram/9.5 calories

DAY 15: EXPERIMENT

Humans truly are creatures of habit. It's easy in life to fall into a routine and do the same things, eat at the same restaurants, prepare the same dishes, and travel to the same places. When our habits bring us some level of pleasure or comfort, we tend to do them even more. Unfortunately, this behavior limits us and keeps us from potentially wonderful experiences that could bring us joy and great memories. Travel habits are a great illustration of this point. People often find a destination that they like and then visit it repeatedly, forsaking the opportunity to try a new locale with its new experiences. The mind is as open as you allow it to be. When you put up barriers, you will exist in those confines. Eating habits are very similar. Many of our culinary preferences are set early in life. We find the flavors and textures and combinations we like and when faced with options, we tend to go back to the known and reliable. For these twenty days you are going to tear down those walls of familiarity and roam uncharted territories. Try new fruits and vegetables or different ways of preparing them. Experiment with some of the recipes in the back of this book. When you visit your favorite restaurant don't order your favorite dish, but give something else a try. Push your exercise and try something new that you might've thought too difficult or not interesting. The world is a vast ocean of opportunity, but unless you explore it, its pleasures will remain hidden. I heard it described best as: "Life begins at the end of your comfort zone."

Breakfast

Choose one of the following:

- Baked Apple Oatmeal Cups (see recipe, page 177)
- Berry Delight Smoothie (see recipe, page 174) or another smoothie that's 350 calories or less

Side (choose one of the following):

- 1 slice 100% whole-grain or 100% whole-wheat toast
- 2 slices turkey bacon

Snack

Choose one of the following:

- Kale chips: ½ cup raw kale (stems removed) baked with 1 teaspoon olive oil at 400 degrees until crisp
- 150 calories or less snack option

Lunch

Choose one of the following:

- Black Bean and Tomato Salad (see recipe, page 199)
- Large green garden salad with 3 ounces chicken or fish and 2 tablespoons salad dressing (see recipes, pages 234 and 235)

Snack

Choose one of the following:

- 1½ cups sugar snap peas (other options: 8 to 10 baby carrots or 1 stalk celery, cut into sections)
- 150 calories or less snack option

Dinner

Choose one of the following:

- Creole Salmon (see recipe, page 229) with ½ cup bok choy and ½ cup corn
- 4 servings cooked vegetables—corn, zucchini, black beans, and watercress—with ½ cup quinoa

Snack (if desired)

- 100 calories or less snack option

Let's Get Physical

- 14,000 steps
- 3 minutes of jog punches (see page 248)
- 3 minutes of ice skaters (see page 243)
- 3 minutes of steam engines (see page 247)
- 3 sets of 10 squats (see page 246)

FOOD FOR THOUGHT
Feel Full Fiber

Fiber is a type of carbohydrate naturally found in food and extremely important for our digestive system. Fruit, vegetables, whole grains, nuts, beans, and legumes are good sources of dietary fiber. The bad news is that many of us are not eating enough of it! The Institute of Medicine recommends 30 to 38 grams a day for men and 25 grams a day for women between eighteen and fifty years old. If a woman is fifty-one and older she should be consuming 21 grams a day. Be careful of the fiber you consume, however, because not all fiber is created equal. Look at the packaging label carefully. Manufacturers often add fiber to foods to boost the fiber levels. Some of the common names include cellulose, inulin, lignin, maltodextrin, pectin, and polydextrose. These added fibers are counted in the food's total fiber count, but they haven't been proven to offer the same health benefits as the natural food fiber. Manufactured or synthetic fiber doesn't provide the vitamins and minerals found in the food sources of fiber, because they are removed during processing. Foods high in dietary fiber also make you feel full, whereas the manufactured fiber may not be as effective at producing this feeling of fullness.

DAY 16: RESTORE

Every second you're awake your body is in a state of stimulation. Whether it's the sound of cars driving by on the street, cold temperatures causing you to shiver and your blood vessels to narrow, or the smell of fresh pizza emanating from a brick oven, one or more of your senses is receiving some type of stimulation. This is why sleep is so important: it's the time your body is the least stimulated and has an opportunity to restore itself. Even if you don't feel tired and look like you're fine, your body is internally fatigued from all that it has to do to keep you alive and performing all of the physical and mental tasks you require of it every day. This entire twenty-day journey is a period of restoration. Imagine you have just finished running a grueling marathon. Your body is not only fatigued, but depleted of electrolytes and fluids. The last thing it wants to do is run another 26.2 miles. It needs time to replenish and reinvigorate. Purging your body of chemicals and artificial ingredients stuffed into all of the processed foods that you are no longer eating will replenish and reinvigorate your cells. Imagine your body getting a chance to rest, rebuild, and reboot. You will feel completely different at the end of this awesome journey!

Breakfast

Choose one of the following:

- Clean Green Smoothie (see recipe, page 172)
- 1½ cups oatmeal; fresh fruit optional

Side (choose one of the following):

- 1 apple, 1 banana, 1 pear, 1 orange, or ½ cup berries
- 1 slice 100% whole-grain or 100% whole-wheat bread

Snack

Choose one of the following:

- 1 cup fruit salad
- 150 calories or less snack option

Lunch

Choose one of the following:

- Whole-Wheat Bruschetta (see recipe, page 197) with small green garden salad
- 1½ cups vegetable, tomato, chicken, lentil, or bean soup with small green garden salad

Snack

Choose one of the following:

- 17 pecans
- 150 calories or less snack option

Dinner

Choose one of the following:

- Deluxe Tuna Tartare (see recipe, page 218) with ½ cup cannellini beans and ½ cup collard greens
- 4 servings vegetables—arugula, squash, eggplant, and broccoli—with 1 cup bean, lentil, or vegetable soup

Snack (if desired)

- 100 calories or less snack option

Let's Get Physical

- 11,000 steps
- 250 jumping jacks (If you have knee problems or can't do a full jumping jack, do a modified jumping jack where you don't have to jump off the ground but rather step to the side instead.)
- 3 minutes of high knees (see page 244)
- 3 minutes of running in place
- 3 minutes of planks (see page 248)

FOOD FOR THOUGHT

Water Wonders

Water is everywhere, but only about 1.1% of the water on earth is suitable to drink. Considering that almost 70% of our body consists of water, we need it in large quantities (at least 6 or more cups per day). Water does everything from preventing your skin from sagging to increasing your mental and physical performance. But many people don't know that water allows the body to metabolize fats more efficiently. Water is essential for your body to function properly and for you to stay alive. One of your most important tasks is to prevent yourself from getting dehydrated. Waiting until you're thirsty before you take a drink is often too late, as it's a sign your body had reached the point of dehydration.

DAY 17: INTRODUCE

"Out with the old and in with the new." It sounds simple, but its impact can be substantial. You have already cleansed yourself and your environment of those old elements that obstructed your path to happiness and success. Now it's time to introduce new things that are going to give you better health and a better quality of life. Our environment impacts us in ways that we are aware of, but also in ways that we don't even know. Surround yourself with the "right" things and the "right" people. You know what foods and beverages you need to succeed for these twenty days, so make sure you have them in proper supply and in the correct locations in *and* out of your house so that you will have them constantly available. Investing in the supplies you need is a direct investment in your success that will pay major dividends. Spending as much time as possible around supportive and positive people is also something that will increase your chances of staying on this healthy journey and reaching your goals. Studies have consistently shown that we have a propensity to model the attitudes and certain attributes of those with whom we spend the most time. Someone else who is trying to improve their life and do better is going to be an inspiration and source of encouragement as you try the same. One study even found that obesity can spread from friend to friend just like a virus. When one person gains weight, his or her close friends tend to gain weight also. It's not just your food environment that matters, but your social network.

Breakfast

Choose one of the following:

- Sweet and Tart Smoothie (see recipe, page 173) or another fruit smoothie (350 calories or less)
- 2 scrambled eggs cooked in extra-virgin olive oil with 1 ounce cheese and your choice of seasonings

Side (choose one of the following):

- 1 slice 100% whole-grain or 100% whole-wheat bread
- 1 piece of fruit or ½ cup berries

Snack

Choose one of the following:

- 1 small baked sweet potato
- 150 calories or less snack option

Lunch

Choose one of the following:

- Chicken, Kale, and Sweet Potato Extravaganza (see recipe, page 201)
- 1 cup whole-wheat pasta with green beans and sun-dried tomatoes

Snack

Choose one of the following:

- 2¼-inch-thick pineapple rounds, grilled or sautéed
- 150 calories or less snack option

Dinner

Choose one of the following:

- Cod with Zucchini Salsa (see recipe, page 219) with ½ cup arugula and ½ cup carrots
- 6 ounces grilled turkey or skinless chicken with ½ cup peas and ½ cup corn

Snack (if desired)

- 100 calories or less snack option

Let's Get Physical

- REST DAY (Still try to complete 8,000 steps or more.)

- - -

FOOD FOR THOUGHT

Sweet with Purpose (Honey)

- - -

The next time you reach for something to sweeten your food, you might want to pause for a second and give serious contemplation to choosing honey. The fact that it can make almost anything taste better is already a well-acknowledged fact. Whereas other sweeteners do very little other than light up the pleasure-reward pathways in your brain, honey contains a host of nutrients, including vitamins B1, B2, B3, B6, and C. Its array of hardy minerals includes calcium, chlorine, iron, phosphate, potassium, and sodium. If you're trying to lose a little weight, try some dissolved in warm water; honey can help in digesting the fat stored in your body. It helps with muscle recuperation after exercise and helps restore glycogen (sugar storage) levels once depleted. And if all of that isn't enough, it promotes rehydration, something that can benefit every cell in your body. Honey does have calories and can raise your insulin levels just like other sweet products, but none of them come with as many nutrients and the potential to improve your health in so many ways.

DAY 18: LEAD

Some leadership is vocal and public, some is quiet and anonymous. One of the best qualities of a leader is leading by example. It sounds like a cliché, but it's very true that actions speak louder than words. You are in the midst of a process that is transformational not only for you, but for others around you, many of whom you may not even realize are paying attention. Many people know what they need to do to live and feel better, but don't or can't find it within themselves to carry out the necessary steps to make it happen. When you ask people about the turning point in their journey to success, they will often say it was something as simple as hearing someone else's inspirational story or witnessing the quiet progress of a neighbor or colleague who through hard work and tenacity accomplished what at one point might've seemed like an unattainable goal. Whether they comment or not, others are watching and taking notes and are inspired by your dedication. When you inspire others to do better and they start making changes in their own lives, not only is it rewarding, but often their response can become another motivating force for you to continue in your journey. You are not responsible for the actions of others, but it can be quite a rewarding experience when you're able to positively influence them.

Breakfast

Choose one of the following:

- Grilled cheese sandwich on 100% whole-grain or 100% whole-wheat bread
- Down-Home Yogurt Parfait (see recipe, page 180)

Side (choose one of the following):

- 1 hard-boiled egg with your preferred seasoning
- ½ cup berries

Snack

Choose one of the following:

- Roasted chickpeas: ½ cup canned chickpeas tossed with 2 tablespoons olive oil, spread on a cookie sheet, and lightly salted; bake at 350 degrees for 12 to 15 minutes
- 150 calories or less snack option

Lunch

Choose one of the following:

- Tomato Chickpea Salad (see recipe, page 196)
- 5-ounce grilled veggie or turkey burger with tomato, lettuce, and 1 ounce cheese on 100% whole-grain bun with small green garden salad

Snack

Choose one of the following:

- 1 large apple, sliced, sprinkled with cinnamon
- 150 calories or less snack option

Dinner

Choose one of the following:

- Super Simple Herb-Encrusted Salmon (see recipe, page 230)
- Large green garden salad with olives and 3 ounces chicken strips or fish

Snack (if desired)

- 100 calories or less snack option

Let's Get Physical

- 15,000 steps
- 7 flights of steps (A trip up and down is considered to be one flight; each flight should have 10 steps or more. See page 246.)
- 3 minutes of running in place
- 3 minutes of ice skaters (see page 243)
- 3 sets of 10 squats (see page 246)

■ ■

FOOD FOR THOUGHT

War and Peace (Calcium)

■ ■

The wonders of calcium and its effects on bone, teeth, nerve signaling, muscle movement, and proper blood vessel function are well known. This essential mineral is simply something our body can't live without. But like any powerful star, calcium has its friends and its enemies. Vitamin D is one of its biggest allies. It helps move calcium through the intestinal tract so that it can be absorbed, and it also triggers the release and circulation of calcium that has been locked up in the bones. On the other side of the battlefield, there are enemies of calcium that reduce its absorption by the body. Too much alcohol, caffeine, or sodium can make calcium difficult to digest and process.

DAY 19: APPRECIATE

Gratitude is an underestimated and underutilized emotion. It's so easy to get lost in the pursuit of goals. Whether it's trying to make a certain amount of money in a year, making the roster of a sporting team, purchasing a particular type of car, or crossing off items on your personal bucket list, we are constantly in search of the next accomplishment. While these goals are important to motivate us and give us purpose, they can also cloud out all of the things we have already accomplished and the gratitude we should have for doing so. A study looked at the happiest people in the world and found the Danes ahead of the pack. One of the major reasons why they are so happy is their gratitude. Their philosophy is simple—what you don't have shouldn't monopolize your thoughts; rather focus on what you *do* have or what you have accomplished. These are things that keep you well grounded and bring joy. Gratitude is not just an act of piety, but has real implications for emotional well-being. Psychologists have done extensive research on gratitude and found that those who are grateful are happier, are more optimistic, and feel better about their lives. Be grateful for even the smallest indicators of progress or goals that you achieve. For example, if you have been someone who can't live without a can of soda or a cup of coffee every day, and you are able to go several days in a row without it, but slip on the fourth day, don't spend your energy on the failing of that fourth day. Think about how great it was that you were able to achieve three consecutive days without your must-have drink. The texture of life is not built on those occasional grand, earth-shattering moments, but on the hundreds of smaller events that come in between them.

Breakfast

Choose one of the following:

- 2 scrambled eggs in extra-virgin olive oil with cheese and peppers
- 6 or 8 ounces low-fat or fat-free organic Greek yogurt parfait

Side (choose one of the following):

- 1 slice 100% whole-grain toast
- 1 piece of fruit or ½ cup berries

Snack

Choose one of the following:

- 1½ strips low-fat string cheese
- 150 calories or less snack option

Lunch

Choose one of the following:

- Turkey and Three Amigos Chili (see recipe, page 221)
- 1 cup whole-wheat pasta with squash and corn

Snack

Choose one of the following:

- Frozen banana slices (1 whole banana)
- 150 calories or less snack option

Dinner

Choose one of the following:

- Sweet Potato Pesto Pasta (see recipe, page 224) with ½ cup pinto beans and ½ cup cauliflower
- Large green garden salad with 2 tablespoons salad dressing (see recipes, pages 234 and 235) and 1 cup bean, lentil, chickpea, or chicken soup

Snack (if desired)

- 100 calories or less snack option

Let's Get Physical

- 18,000 steps
- 200 jumping jacks (If you have knee problems or can't do a full jumping jack, do a modified jumping jack where you don't have to jump off the ground but rather step to the side instead.)
- 3 minutes of jog punches (see page 248)
- 3 minutes of planks (see page 248)
- 3 minutes of steam engines (see page 247)

FOOD FOR THOUGHT

Ginger Greatness

Ginger's gastronomic contributions are well known and much enjoyed. But that knobby, eccentric-looking root does more than spice up your stir-fry or hot tea. Ginger is a natural anti-inflammatory and has been used for thousands of years in China to treat pain. Recent studies have also shown that ginger is an effective pain reliever, particularly for conditions such as arthritis. Beyond pain, ginger has also been shown to be helpful at relieving headaches, menstrual cramps, muscle soreness, and nausea. One more surprise: when the temperature dips, a shot of ginger might help your blood circulation keep you warm.

DAY 20: THRIVE

You have spent the last nineteen days undergoing a wonderful transformation physically, emotionally, and mentally. It might not have been the easiest time and there were likely moments when you wanted to end your mission and return to those convenient processed foods and sugary drinks. Were you perfect? Probably not. But you've made it to the end and that's what really counts. These twenty days have been all about opening your mind to new things, gaining confidence, developing a better relationship with your body, better understanding how far you can push yourself, and finding joy in the power of transformation. Your body has been reinvigorated with all of the superfoods, antioxidants, vitamins, minerals, and other phytonutrients you've carefully fed it. It's had a chance to reset and free itself from the toxic by-products of processed foods and chemical-laden drinks. Don't throw all of these hard-earned gains away and return to your old habits. You were never asked to be perfect at any time during these twenty days, and you're not expected to be perfect going forward. But after all of this work and determination, it *is* expected that you take the lessons you've learned and apply them to the rest of your life so you not just survive, but *thrive*!

Breakfast

Choose one of the following:

- Omelet made with 2 eggs and ¼ cup diced veggies
- 1 cup oatmeal with sliced fruit

Side (choose one of the following):

- 2 slices turkey bacon
- 1 apple, 1 orange, or ½ grapefruit

Snack

Choose one of the following:

- Loaded pepper slices: 1 cup red bell pepper slices topped with ¼ cup warm black beans and 1 tablespoon guacamole or 1 tablespoon diced avocado
- 150 calories or less snack option

Lunch

Choose one of the following:

- Turkey or chicken sandwich on 100% whole-grain or 100% whole-wheat bread with small green garden salad
- Large green garden salad with 2 tablespoons salad dressing, olives (optional) and 3 ounces chicken or fish

Snack

Choose one of the following:

- 10 walnut halves and 1 sliced kiwi
- 150 calories or less snack option

Dinner

Choose one of the following:

- 6 oz grilled, skinless, boneless chicken breast with ½ cup brown rice and ½ cup black beans
- 4 servings cooked vegetables (black beans, carrots, cabbage, cauliflower) with 1 cup bean, lentil, chickpea, or chicken soup

Snack (if desired)

- 100 calories or less snack option

Let's Get Physical

- REST DAY (Still try to complete 8,000 steps or more.)

■ ■

FOOD FOR THOUGHT

Homemade Is Best Made

■ ■

Cooking can be intimidating, especially if it's something that you've arrived at later in lfe. But taking an approach that's curious rather than too serious can make all the difference in the world when it comes to enjoying the experience. Making your own meals and snacks is beneficial for other reasons too. First, it actually can save money. At a restaurant, you're paying for more than just the food. The restaurant owner needs to pay employees and various bills, and that can only be done by charging you more and making a profit. Second, you are in control of the food environment. You know exactly what you're putting into the food, unlike what happens with commercially prepared foods whose quantities of fat, salt, and sugar are unknown to you. Third, you can save lots of time. When you plan ahead, a home-cooked meal saves you time from ordering, driving to the restaurant to pick it up, then returning home to eat it. There are plenty of recipes that take no more than 30 minutes to prepare. Last, cooking and eating at home is an opportunity for family to gather around the stove and table and share. In this fast-paced, digital-dominant world, we are so plugged into things that keep us separate. Cooking a homemade meal and sitting down and enjoying it with your family is a perfect and fun occasion to come together!

six

Reemergence

Congrats on completing twenty clean days. Did you have some challenges along the way, either large or small? Did you achieve any results? If so, were these results external or internal or both? Have you developed a new mind-set around eating and moving healthier? These are important questions to ask and answer, as they will give you better insight into your journey and context for moving forward. So what's next? Is it possible for you to continue to eat clean for the rest of your life? Absolutely. You now know what it means to eat clean and all of the health-boosting nutrients processed foods are lacking. Switching from a heavily processed diet to one that is predominantly clean has likely caused your energy and mood levels to be improved.

Are you going to eat perfectly clean for the rest of your life? Probably not. You are going to want to eat some of those fun foods you've missed over the last few weeks—maybe some chocolate chip cookies, some pancakes, or some french fries. Don't feel bad about this! The purpose of the Clean 20 is to help you hit the reset button. It was not meant to deprive you of having some of the fun you find in processed foods. It's not a matter of *if* you will add back some of the foods and beverages that didn't make your Clean 20 list; it's a matter of *when* and *how*.

It's time to reintroduce these foods, but reintroduce them so you don't unwind all the progress you've made over the last twenty days. Be respectful of your transformation and the positive impact the Clean 20 reset has had on your body. Your preferences have been altered since you have been avoiding a lot of the processed ingredients and the chemicals that they contain. Even your digestive system has been reset to expect a different quality and quantity of food. So it's important to take it slow and not rush back to indulging in all of those old foods at once; otherwise you will find your stomach getting a little upset, your mood and energy levels changing, and your movements a little sluggish.

As you prepare to reintroduce foods, the hope is that eating clean for the last twenty days has encouraged you to keep some foods and beverages on a "permanently banned" list. Which and how many items make this list is completely up to you. But foods loaded with artificial coloring, heaps of added sugars, and high-fructose corn syrup will hopefully make this list very quickly. So now it's time to make two lists. The first is your permanently banned items that you will decide never to eat again or to consume rarely. The other list is comprised of the food items that weren't allowed for the last twenty days, but that you would like to slowly reintroduce into your diet.

This is what the lists might look like:

Once you have your two lists made up, you are ready to start to reemerge. This reemergence period is also twenty days. The idea is that every two or three days, you should reintroduce one item into your diet. This means that by the end of this reemergence period, you will be predominantly eating cleaner foods, but you will also be able to eat other foods that may not be the healthiest, but that you still enjoy.

The next thing for you to try is splitting the difference between the lists. You should attempt to create some alternatives to some of the really unhealthy foods that taste so

BANNED
Soda
Potato chips
BBQ sauce containing high-fructose corn syrup
Cotton candy
Fried fish
Donuts
Iced tea with lots of sugar and artificial ingredients

REINTRODUCED
Pizza
Beef cheeseburger
Steak
Chocolate chip cookies
Pancakes and waffles
Beef empanadas
Tortilla chips and salsa

good to you. You might also try to reduce the volume of the processed food and add a clean food item to make up for the calorie hole you now have with this reduction. For example, if you are accustomed to eating oil-popped popcorn loaded with butter and salt, try an air-popped popcorn that's lightly tossed in sea salt. Instead of drinking soda, try some flavored fizzy water or make it yourself by squeezing citrus juice into a glass of seltzer water. The idea is that while you are not expected to eat perfectly, your overall food and drink choices will be elevated to a higher level of healthiness.

How often can you do The Clean 20 Daily Meal Plan? As often as you like. Why not? This plan is full of healthy, nutritious food, close to the way nature has provided it to us. This style of eating should be the norm and not the exception. The fact that we have to work and sacrifice to eat healthy is a testament to how badly we have things out of order. It shouldn't take extra effort to do what should be natural and beneficial.

Now that you've done the entire twenty days, you also are aware that doing just some of them can be a benefit also. Try an abbreviated version where you go on the plan for only seven or ten days. Think of it the way you would think about taking your car to the mechanic to get a tune-up. Getting all of your fluid levels topped off as well as your engine and brakes checked is important to make sure you either catch a problem before it's too damaging and costly or prevent a problem from happening in the first place. You are getting your mind and body tuned up to feel and look their best and to be prepared to deliver peak performance.

Part III

The Bonus

seven

■ ■ ■ ■ ■ ■ ■ ■ ■ ■ ■ ■ ■ ■ ■ ■

The Clean 20 Recipes

These recipes are based on the Clean 20 guidelines. Some of the ingredients may not be on your original Clean 20 list, but that is all right. Remember, you're allowed to add more clean ingredients if you desire. There also is no rule about when you use these recipes during your day. If you want to cook a dinner recipe at lunch and vice versa, that's not a problem. These recipes are really a guide, not something that is rigid and shouldn't be changed. The idea is for you to experiment with new foods and combinations and flavors. As long as you're using approved clean ingredients, feel free to play with them and make substitutions. Most important, open your mind to the intoxicating pleasure of new foods and have lots of *fun*!

BREAKFAST

Clean Green Smoothie

Sweet and Tart Smoothie

Berry Delight Smoothie

Baby Spinach Omelet

Easy Egg Frittata

Baked Apple Oatmeal Cups

Egg and Turkey Casserole

Down-Home Yogurt Parfait

Nifty Bacon, Egg, and Cheese Sandwich

Energy Explosion Yogurt

Heavenly Blueberry Oatmeal

Baked Oatmeal

CLEAN GREEN SMOOTHIE

A sweet green smoothie is the best of two worlds. The sweetness excites the palate, while the vegetable and fruit exhilarate your cells and tissues that use their phytonutrients to carry out life's daily functions. This is a wake-me-up smoothie that doesn't disappoint.

Serves 2, Serving size: 12 ounces

2 Gala apples, peeled, cored, and sliced
1 ripe banana, peeled and sliced
¾ cup green seedless grapes
½ cup chilled unsweetened almond milk
¼ teaspoon ground cinnamon
½ cup packed curly kale, stems removed

Combine all ingredients with ½ cup ice in a blender and puree until smooth. Enjoy.

SWEET AND TART SMOOTHIE

This smoothie is full of contrasting flavors that satisfy you and load you up with powerhouse nutrients from the spinach and flaxseed. The sweetness of the banana and orange juice might swallow the earthy taste of the spinach, but they can't stop it from delivering an impressive array of phytonutrients.

Serves 2, Serving size: 12 ounces

1 cup loosely packed baby spinach, stems removed

½ cup organic low-fat or nonfat plain Greek yogurt

½ cup fresh orange juice

1 ripe banana, peeled and sliced

½ small lemon, peeled, sliced into sections, and seeded

½ small lime, peeled, sliced into sections, and seeded

2 tablespoons unfiltered organic flaxseed oil (optional)

Combine all ingredients in a blender with 7 ice cubes and puree until smooth.

BERRY DELIGHT SMOOTHIE

There's nothing like starting your day with a cup full of anti-oxidants and a powerful vitamin concoction to boost energy levels as you prepare for the day ahead. In less than five minutes you'll have enough to fill you up on your way out the door and get all the nutrition you need to keep you going.

Serves 2, Serving size: 12 ounces

2 cups mixed berries
1 banana, peeled and sliced
1 cup organic low-fat or nonfat
   plain Greek yogurt

1 cup unsweetened almond milk
½ teaspoon organic honey
6 ice cubes

Combine ingredients in a blender and puree until smooth.

BABY SPINACH OMELET

This versatile recipe takes less than ten minutes to prepare and gives you plenty of opportunity to choose a filling you prefer. Spinach and cheese complete the mission in this preparation, but don't be afraid to experiment with other tasty combinations.

Serves 1

2 eggs
⅛ teaspoon grated nutmeg
¼ teaspoon onion powder
2 tablespoons water

Salt and freshly ground black pepper
1 cup baby spinach leaves
1 tablespoon extra-virgin olive oil
1 ounce cheddar cheese

1. In a bowl, beat eggs, nutmeg, onion powder, water, and salt and pepper, then stir in spinach.

2. Heat oil in a small nonstick skillet over medium-high heat, making sure you tilt pan to coat bottom.

3. Pour egg mixture into skillet. Edges should firm up immediately.

4. Gently push the cooked portions from the edges toward the center with a spatula, allowing the uncooked eggs to come in contact with the hot skillet surface. Continue to tilt pan while gently moving the cooked portion back and forth.

5. When the top surface of the eggs is firm and there's no visible uncooked egg, place the cheese on one side of the omelet. Fold it in half with spatula. Let it cook for another minute, then flip and cook the other side for another minute.

6. Add salt and pepper to taste and serve hot.

EASY EGG FRITTATA

This frittata may be easy to make, but that doesn't mean it's a lightweight in what it delivers. Beyond the burst of flavor, it also brings along lots of nutrients such as vitamin A, vitamin D, calcium, choline, and a respectable amount of protein. In less than fifteen minutes you'll have what it takes to get your day off to a good start!

Serves 2

4 eggs
¼ cup 1% or fat-free milk
¼ teaspoon dried thyme
Salt and freshly ground black
  pepper

3 turkey bacon slices, cooked
  and diced
3 ounces cheddar or feta cheese
1 tablespoon extra-virgin olive oil

1. Beat eggs, milk, thyme, and salt and pepper in medium bowl until blended. Add bacon and cheese and mix well.

2. Heat oil in an 8-inch skillet over medium heat. When hot, pour in egg mixture. After 2 minutes, lower heat and cook for 8 minutes, or until eggs are almost set.

3. Remove skillet from heat. Cover and let stand until eggs are completely cooked and set (5 to 10 minutes).

4. Cut into wedges, season with salt and pepper to taste, and serve warm.

BAKED APPLE OATMEAL CUPS

This simple recipe combines two popular breakfast items and melds them together to create a dish that has the earthy goodness of whole grains and the natural sweetness of baked apples. The beauty of this recipe is that you can have fun and add berries or other ingredients to the apple cup and have a different gastronomic experience each time you make it.

Serves 2

1 cup old-fashioned rolled oats
1 cup organic unsweetened
    almond milk
¼ teaspoon organic honey
½ teaspoon cinnamon

2 large red apples (try Honeycrisp
    or Braeburn if you can)
1 tablespoon chopped walnuts
    (optional)
Juice of ½ lemon

1. Preheat oven to 350 degrees.

2. Mix oats, almond milk, honey, cinnamon, and lemon juice in a small bowl, and set aside for 20 minutes.

3. Cut the top off the apples and remove their cores.

4. Use a spoon to hollow the apple so that the oatmeal filling can fit.

5. Mix the oatmeal with the nuts if you choose to use them and fill the apples until the cavity is full.

6. Place the apples in a baking dish and add approximately ¼ inch hot water to the pan. Cover with foil and bake for 30 to 40 minutes, until apples are tender but not mushy.

7. Serve warm.

EGG AND TURKEY CASSEROLE

The combination of eggs and turkey in the morning is a great way to replenish your energy and restore important levels of protein, iron, vitamins A, E, and B12, and choline, which can be further depleted while you're sleeping. Hardy enough to satisfy your hunger, but also light enough so that you don't feel weighed down as you start your day, this dish does everything a good breakfast should do.

Serves 4

2 teaspoons olive oil
1 pound ground turkey
¼ teaspoon chili powder
½ teaspoon salt
½ teaspoon pepper
5 eggs

1 small sweet potato
¾ cup kale leaves, stems removed
7 ripe cherry tomatoes, halved
¼ cup fresh basil leaves,
    finely chopped

1. Preheat the oven to 375 degrees.

2. Grease an 8-inch square baking dish with 1 teaspoon oil.

3. Put 1 teaspoon oil in a medium-sized skillet and add the turkey. Chop it up into small bits so more surface area of the meat is exposed to the pan. Cook over medium-high heat until browned through. Add chili powder and half of the salt and pepper.

4. Beat the eggs in a bowl and season with remaining salt and pepper.

5. Peel the sweet potato and slice into thin discs.

6. Arrange the potato slices on the bottom of the pan, then spread the cooked turkey on top. Next, layer on the kale evenly, then pour the eggs on top. Finally, layer on the tomatoes and basil.

7. Place dish in the oven and cook for 35 to 45 minutes, until cooked through.

8. Serve hot.

DOWN-HOME YOGURT PARFAIT

Not everyone wants to eat a big, complicated breakfast or has the time to put together a multi-step meal during a hectic morning. This yogurt parfait is something that you can whip together in less than five minutes and still have the taste and satisfaction of a meal that might've taken half an hour. And the bonus? You can take it with you to go.

Serves 1

¼ cup blueberries
1 cup organic low-fat or nonfat
    plain Greek yogurt
2 tablespoons granola

¼ cup sliced banana
¼ cup sliced strawberries
½ teaspoon organic honey
    (optional)

1. Put blueberries into a glass that is larger than 8 ounces.

2. Scoop ½ cup yogurt onto the berries.

3. Add half of the granola in a layer on top of the yogurt.

4. Add banana slices on top of the granola.

5. Add the rest of the yogurt.

6. Add the remaining granola.

7. Top with the sliced strawberries and drizzle with honey if desired.

NIFTY BACON, EGG, AND CHEESE SANDWICH

This classic breakfast sandwich is even better when you make it at home rather than picking it up at the drive-thru. Not only is it fresher, but it's also healthier. Full of protein and whole grains, this is a great way to boost your energy levels and get your day off to a strong start.

Serves 1

2 slices turkey bacon
2 slices 100% whole-wheat or 100% whole-grain bread, toasted
2 eggs

Salt and freshly ground black pepper
1 tablespoon shredded cheese
2 tomato slices

1. Cook bacon in a nonstick skillet over medium heat until cooked through. Arrange on one slice of toast.

2. Beat eggs with salt and pepper, then add to the skillet and cook until the edges are set. Flip and add the shredded cheese and cook for another 30 to 60 seconds.

3. Fold the egg on top of the bacon, then top with the tomato slices. Season with salt and pepper to taste, then add the second slice of toast to complete the sandwich.

4. Serve warm.

ENERGY EXPLOSION YOGURT

There's nothing like starting the day with a combination of fresh flavors that will tingle your senses and restore your energy. The steadiness of oats combines with the explosive sweetness of fruit and honey. Antioxidants are practically jumping out of this dish ready to get you going for the day.

Serves 1

One 5.3-ounce container plain
   nonfat organic Greek yogurt
½ teaspoon organic honey
¼ teaspoon cinnamon
2 tablespoons rolled oats
Grated zest of 1 lemon

2 tablespoons dried blueberries
   (or dried cranberries or other
   berries; optional)
1 teaspoon almonds, halved
   (optional)

1. In a small bowl, combine yogurt, honey, cinnamon, oats, and lemon zest and stir to mix. Let stand about 5 minutes to soften oats.

2. Sprinkle blueberries and almonds over the top and enjoy.

HEAVENLY BLUEBERRY OATMEAL

This modern twist on a traditional recipe delivers big waves of flavor while increasing the already huge burst of nutrition naturally found in the whole grains of oats. Easy to make either on the stove or in the microwave, this breakfast cereal recipe is one you might want to enjoy any time of the day.

Serves 2

1 cup old-fashioned rolled oats
1⅓ cups water
1 teaspoon organic honey
¼ teaspoon cinnamon
¼ teaspoon ground nutmeg
Pinch of salt

⅓ cup blueberries
½ cup low-fat milk, soy milk, or unsweetened almond milk
½ teaspoon finely chopped or grated orange zest

1. Put oatmeal, water, honey, cinnamon, nutmeg, and salt in a large microwave-safe mixing bowl. Cover the bowl with a plate or wet paper towel. Microwave on high for 3 to 5 minutes.

2. Let sit for a couple of minutes, then remove cover. Stir in blueberries, milk, and orange zest.

3. Cover bowl again and cook in microwave for another 2 to 3 minutes. Let sit for 1 minute before eating.

BAKED OATMEAL

Most people are accustomed to their oatmeal being prepared
on top of the stove or in the microwave, but if time permits, a
true delight is having it cooked in the oven. Baking allows the
oats and other ingredients to fully reach and blend their peak
flavors. Rich and savory, the taste is only equaled by the large
amount of nutrition in each bite.

Serves 4

3 cups rolled oats
2 teaspoons ground cinnamon
½ teaspoon salt
1 cup organic low-fat or fat-free
   milk
2 eggs

2 teaspoons organic vanilla
   extract
½ cup melted organic butter
½ cup dried organic cranberries or
   blueberries (optional)

1. Preheat oven to 375°.

2. In a large bowl, mix together oats, cinnamon, and salt. Beat in
milk, eggs, vanilla extract, and melted butter.

3. Stir in dried cranberries or blueberries if desired. Spread into
a 9×13-inch glass baking dish.

4. Bake for 30–35 minutes.

5. Serve hot.

LUNCH

Whole-Wheat Spaghetti with Edamame Pesto Gusto

Chilly Cucumber Soup

Pesto Chicken Salad

Sumptuous Butternut Squash Soup

Turkey Salad

Yummy Baked Tomatoes

Tomato Chickpea Salad

Whole-Wheat Bruschetta

Tomato Puree

Black Bean and Tomato Salad

Succulent Turkey Burger

Chicken, Kale, and Sweet Potato Extravaganza

Avocado and Chickpea Salad

Juicy Chicken Burger

Effortless Kale Chips

Turkey Meatballs

Georgia Peach Salmon

Baked Sweet Potato Fries

WHOLE-WHEAT SPAGHETTI WITH EDAMAME PESTO GUSTO

This recipe is deceptively delicious. You might not be impressed by the individual ingredients, but when you add them together, they make nothing short of culinary magic. Instead of the classic basil, this recipe substitutes edamame, rich in vitamins, protein, and fiber. This delivers a sauce with a hint of earthiness and dash of brightness that puts a healthy spin on traditional Italian cooking.

Serves 4

1 cup frozen shelled edamame, thawed
2 cloves garlic, chopped
¼ cup sliced almonds, toasted
¼ cup fresh flat-leaf parsley leaves
Grated zest of ½ lemon

½ cup freshly grated parmesan cheese, plus more for garnish
¼ cup extra-virgin olive oil, plus more as needed
Salt and freshly ground black pepper
1 pound whole-wheat spaghetti

1. Combine edamame, garlic, and almonds in the bowl of a food processor and pulse until finely chopped. Add parsley, lemon zest, parmesan, and oil and pulse until well combined and the edamame is very finely chopped. Transfer the pesto to a large mixing bowl and season with salt and pepper to taste.

2. Bring a large pot of water to a boil and salt it generously. Boil the pasta according to the instructions on the package. Just

before draining, pour 2 or 3 tablespoons of the pasta cooking water into the bowl with the pesto and stir it to loosen.

3. Drain the pasta and transfer it to the pesto bowl and toss with tongs until well coated. Divide the pasta among four serving plates and serve with more parmesan.

CHILLY CUCUMBER SOUP

Cucumber is a vegetable that's perfect for a cold soup. Light, full of water, and relatively neutral in taste, cucumber soup is a great addition to any meal. With little effort and few ingredients, there's not much fuss involved in this creation—and that's exactly the way it should be.

Serves 6

3 cucumbers, halved, peeled, seeds scraped out with a spoon, diced
Sea salt to taste
1 cup organic free-range chicken broth
2 cups organic low-fat buttermilk
2 cups organic low-fat plain Greek yogurt

2 tablespoons chopped fresh dill
1 clove garlic
3 tablespoons fresh lemon juice
½ cup chopped fresh flat-leaf parsley
5 scallions, chopped
¼ cup extra-virgin olive oil
Salt and freshly ground pepper

1. Sprinkle cucumbers with 1 teaspoon salt and let stand for 10 to 15 minutes.

2. Put broth, buttermilk, yogurt, cucumbers, dill, garlic, lemon juice, parsley, scallions, oil, and salt and pepper to taste in a blender or food processor and puree until smooth.

3. Refrigerate for 1 hour and serve cold.

PESTO CHICKEN SALAD

Pesto chicken is wonderful in any preparation and remains just as amazing in salad. The usual ingredient suspects are here, plus a little bit of relish to make what is already a delicious combination taste even better. Eat it alone, on bread, or as a dip; it remains reliably remarkable.

Serves 4

FOR THE PESTO SAUCE:

2 cups fresh basil leaves, stems removed

2 large cloves garlic

3 tablespoons pine nuts

½ cup freshly grated parmesan cheese

Salt and freshly ground pepper

⅓ cup extra-virgin olive oil

FOR THE SALAD:

2 cups shredded hormone-free, pasture-raised rotisserie chicken meat, skin removed

⅓ cup Clean Mayonnaise (see recipe, page 233)

1 tablespoon sweet relish

1 celery stalk, finely diced

2 tablespoons finely chopped red onion

Pepper to taste

8 slices ripe tomato (optional for sandwich)

100% whole-wheat or 100% whole-grain bread (optional for sandwich)

FOR THE PESTO SAUCE:

1. Combine basil, garlic, pine nuts, and parmesan in a food processor and season with salt and pepper to taste.

2. Add the oil slowly while the motor is running. Once emulsified, set aside.

FOR THE SALAD:

1. In a large bowl, stir together chicken, pesto sauce, mayonnaise, relish, celery, and onion and stir well. Season with pepper to taste.

2. Serve as a salad or dip or make into a wrap or sandwich using tomatoes and bread.

SUMPTUOUS BUTTERNUT SQUASH SOUP

Butternut squash soup might be one of most underestimated soups in history. Its rich flavor and smooth texture as well as its full aroma make this dish wonderful any time of the year. You can have enough of it to be your complete meal or consume a smaller portion as an appetizer. Let the aroma fill your nose before you taste. Enjoy the complete experience.

Serves 6

2 tablespoons organic butter
1 red onion, chopped
1 large clove garlic, minced
½ teaspoon grated nutmeg
1 cup cubed peeled Gala or Fuji apple
2 pounds butternut squash, peeled and seeded

3 cups organic vegetable stock mixed with 3 tablespoons extra-virgin olive oil
1 teaspoon ground cumin
¼ cup organic buttermilk
Salt and freshly ground black pepper

1. In a large saucepan or pot, melt butter over medium heat and add onion and garlic. Sauté until soft, about 5 minutes. Sprinkle nutmeg on the apple and add to saucepan.

2. Cut squash into 1-inch chunks.

3. Add squash, stock, and cumin to the saucepan and bring to a simmer, cooking until squash is tender, 10 to 15 minutes.

4. Transfer squash chunks and buttermilk to a food processor or blender and puree until smooth.

5. Return blended squash to pot. Stir and let simmer over low heat for approximately 5 minutes and season with salt and pepper to taste.

TURKEY SALAD

This recipe takes a traditional salad preparation and tweaks it a little to accommodate the succulent turkey meat. The nuts and celery give it a nice crunch, and the homemade Clean Mayonnaise serves not only as a binder, but a contributor of flavor that keeps everything together.

Serves 4

12 ounces turkey cutlets
¼ teaspoon salt
Freshly ground black pepper
Extra-virgin olive oil in a
    spray bottle
½ cup water
2 stalks celery, sliced
1 cup red seedless grapes, halved
¼ cup chopped walnuts, toasted

2 tablespoons chopped fresh
    flat-leaf parsley
4 scallions, sliced
1 tablespoon Clean Mayonnaise
    (see recipe, page 233)
3 tablespoons organic low-fat or
    nonfat plain yogurt
1 teaspoon organic honey
4 leaves Bibb lettuce, for serving

1. Season turkey cutlets with salt, and a sprinkling of pepper.

2. Spray medium-sized nonstick skillet with oil and heat over medium heat. Add turkey and cook until browned, 3 to 4 minutes. Flip the turkey and cook until underside is golden, about 3 minutes more.

3. Pour in the water, reduce heat to medium-low, cover the pan, and cook until turkey is completely cooked through, 6 to 8 minutes more. Remove the turkey from the skillet and let stand until cool.

4. In a medium bowl, toss the celery, grapes, walnuts, parsley, and scallions together until combined.

5. In a small bowl, whisk together the mayonnaise, yogurt, and honey. Using two forks, shred the turkey cutlets and add them to the bowl with the celery and grapes, add the dressing, and toss until well coated and thoroughly mixed.

6. Divide turkey salad among lettuce leaves and serve.

YUMMY BAKED TOMATOES

Full of the antioxidant lycopene, as well as vitamin C, potassium, beta-carotene, and fiber, tomatoes give as much in nutrition as they do in their rich flavor. They are open to a variety of seasonings as well as cooking methods. This simple recipe requires few ingredients and just a little patience before you savor the wonderful combination of flavors.

Serves 4

2 tablespoons olive oil, plus a little more for drizzling
3 cloves garlic, minced
½ teaspoon sea salt
½ teaspoon organic honey
1 teaspoon dried basil
¼ cup freshly grated parmesan cheese
Pinch of red pepper flakes
3 tablespoons water
2 pounds plum tomatoes, halved lengthwise and seeded

1. Preheat the oven to 450 degrees. Line a baking pan with foil.

2. In a large bowl, whisk together the oil, garlic, salt, honey, basil, parmesan, red pepper flakes, and water. Add the tomatoes and toss to coat.

3. Place the tomatoes, cut side up, on the foil and bake for 20 minutes.

4. Drizzle with a splash of olive oil, then serve.

TOMATO CHICKPEA SALAD

The vastly different flavors of the two major ingredients in this salad don't fight each other; rather, they do a culinary tango that's pleasing to the palate. The nutty, satisfying flavor of chickpeas blended with the sweet robust flavor of tomatoes is bridged by the cucumbers and Swiss cheese. Simple yet elegant, this salad is one you'll come back to often.

Serves 4

FOR THE DRESSING:

1 clove of garlic, minced

¼ cup balsamic vinegar

2 tablespoons extra-virgin olive oil

Salt and freshly ground black pepper

FOR THE SALAD:

¾ cup cubed cheddar or Monterey Jack cheese

One 16-ounce can chickpeas, rinsed and drained

1 cup chopped cucumber

2 tablespoons chopped fresh flat-leaf parsley

3 tomatoes, chopped

1 scallion, chopped

Freshly ground black pepper

Sea salt

FOR THE DRESSING:

1. In a small bowl, whisk together garlic, oil, vinegar, and salt and pepper to taste.

FOR THE SALAD:

1. In a large bowl, combine cheese, chickpeas, cucumber, parsley, tomatoes, and scallion.

2. Toss salad with dressing. Cover and refrigerate for at least 1 hour.

3. Season with salt and pepper, to taste, and serve chilled or at room temperature.

WHOLE-WHEAT BRUSCHETTA

This classic Italian dish will never be a wrong choice. You can eat it as a snack or serve it as an appetizer. You can even make an entire meal of it. The trick is to make sure the bread is crusty but not too hard. The mozzarella adds another flavor and more protein to complete this mouthwatering dish.

Makes 10 pieces

5 ripe plum tomatoes, chopped
2 cloves garlic, minced
8 fresh basil leaves, chopped
½ teaspoon sea salt
½ teaspoon pepper

2 tablespoons extra-virgin olive oil
1 loaf 100% whole-wheat or whole-grain bread, sliced ¾ inch thick
1 ounce mozzarella cheese, shredded

1. In a small bowl, combine tomatoes, garlic, basil, salt, and pepper; toss, then set aside.

2. Preheat oven to 450 degrees with rack at the highest slot in the oven.

3. Coat a large baking sheet with oil and arrange the bread slices in a single layer. Brush the top of each piece of bread with oil.

4. Place bread in the oven and bake until it's lightly toasted, 1 to 2 minutes.

5. Remove bread from the oven and spoon the tomato mixture on the oil side, which is facing up. Top each piece with a sprinkle of mozzarella and return bread to oven. Bake for 30 seconds or until cheese melts, but doesn't burn.

6. Remove bread from oven, let cool, then serve.

TOMATO PUREE

This simple puree is perfect when making a tomato soup, casserole, or pasta sauce. It's easy to make, requires few ingredients, and can be prepared in a matter of minutes. This dish is widely produced and used in Mediterranean countries. Once added to dishes, it gives them a bright color and distinctive tomato flavor.

Makes approximately 1 quart

2 pounds ripe plum tomatoes

1. Run the tomatoes under cool water and pat try.

2. Peel the tomatoes, then halve them and trim soft spots or other imperfections.

3. Remove the core and scrape out seeds and watery pulp.

4. Coarsely chop the tomatoes.

5. Fill a deep pan with water and bring to a boil over medium heat; once boiling, put in the tomatoes, reduce heat to medium-low, and simmer until they've released some of their juices and are tender, 8 to 10 minutes.

6. Remove tomatoes from hot water and place in cold water for 3 minutes.

7. Place tomatoes in a blender or food processor and puree until smooth.

BLACK BEAN AND TOMATO SALAD

There are some dishes that simply aren't meant to be the star; rather, they shine in a supporting role. This salad plays that role perfectly and is a great companion to a grilled chicken breast or fish fillet. The lime and cilantro brighten the dish and make it memorable.

Serves 4

2 Hass avocados, diced
5 fresh basil leaves, finely chopped
One 15-ounce can black beans,
   rinsed and drained
2 tablespoons minced fresh cilantro
1 seedless cucumber, peeled
   and diced

1 small yellow onion, minced
Juice of 1 lime
3 ripe plum tomatoes, diced
Sea salt and freshly ground
   black pepper

1. Combine all ingredients and mix well, seasoning with salt and pepper to taste.

2. Refrigerate and serve chilled.

SUCCULENT TURKEY BURGER

Why should beef have all the fun when turkey can be equally tasty and supply almost the same amount of protein? This simple burger is juicy, satisfying, and full of flavor. In less than fifteen minutes you'll be biting into your creation, amazed at how a few ingredients and a few spices could deliver such gratification.

Serves 4

1 pound ground turkey
2 tablespoons extra-virgin olive oil
1 tablespoon organic
    Worcestershire sauce
½ teaspoon salt

¼ teaspoon black pepper
1 ounce cheddar cheese (for
    each burger)
1 large slice tomato (for each burger)

1. In a large mixing bowl, knead together turkey, ½ tablespoon oil, Worcestershire sauce, salt, and pepper, making sure ingredients are mixed well.

2. Divide meat into four equal patties.

3. Heat a large skillet over medium heat and pour remaining oil in to coat the entire surface.

4. Cook burgers, flipping on both sides until desired temperature. Place cheese on the burgers a few minutes before it's finished so that it softens and melts.

5. Serve salad style or on a whole-grain bun with tomato.

CHICKEN, KALE, AND SWEET POTATO EXTRAVAGANZA

This dish of eclectic flavors and textures makes what would be an otherwise boring breast of chicken exciting to the palate. The protein, fiber, vitamins, and other nutrients are available to you for a relatively paltry amount of calories. It won't take much to fill you up and make you feel good.

Serves 2

1 large bunch of kale, stems removed

¼ teaspoon ground cumin

3 cloves garlic, minced

2 tablespoons extra-virgin olive oil

Sea salt and freshly ground black pepper

1 large sweet potato, peeled and cubed

Two 6-ounce boneless, skinless chicken breasts

½ cup grape tomatoes, halved

Juice of ½ large lemon

2 cups mixed salad greens

1. Preheat oven to 400 degrees.

2. In a large bowl, toss the kale with the cumin, garlic, 1 tablespoon oil, ¼ teaspoon salt, and pepper to taste.

3. Add cubed sweet potato to a large baking sheet. Add kale mixture to the baking sheet and toss. Roast until potatoes are softened and kale is crisp, 15 to 20 minutes.

4. Flatten chicken breasts to about ½-inch thick, then place in oil-coated baking pan. Season with salt and pepper.

5. Return kale mixture to large bowl, adding tomatoes, lemon juice, 1 tablespoon oil, salad greens, and salt and pepper to taste.

6. Plate the chicken and kale salad. Serve warm.

AVOCADO AND CHICKPEA SALAD

This simple recipe is full of protein and fiber. Easy to make with a rich flavor that isn't dominated by the avocado, the simple dressing really makes the difference. You can eat this alone or use it to complement a fish or chicken dish.

Serves 2

2 tablespoons chopped fresh cilantro
Juice of ½ lemon
¼ cup olive oil
1 tablespoon organic mustard
⅛ teaspoon black pepper
¼ teaspoon sea salt

1 Hass avocado, chunked
One 15-ounce can chickpeas, rinsed and drained
½ small red onion, thinly sliced
2 cups kale leaves, stems removed
2 cups arugula

1. In a large bowl, whisk together cilantro, lemon juice, oil, mustard, pepper and salt.

2. Add avocado, chickpeas, onion, and mixed greens to oil mixture and toss well.

3. Serve at room temperature.

JUICY CHICKEN BURGER

This twist on the classic burger brings a powerful bonus of flavor and nutrition. Substituting chicken for beef doesn't come at much of a cost. You get almost the same amount of protein, but you consume less fat and fewer calories, and you pick up significant amounts of vitamins B3 and B6. This quick and tidy recipe will be a welcome addition to your burger arsenal.

Serves 2

1 tablespoon extra-virgin olive oil
1 pound ground chicken
   (or turkey)
1 clove garlic, minced
½ teaspoon ground cumin
½ small yellow onion, finely chopped
1 teaspoon Clean Mayonnaise
   (see recipe, page 233)
½ teaspoon paprika

¼ cup finely shredded cheddar
   cheese
Sea salt and freshly ground black
   pepper
Lettuce
1 slice of tomato (for each burger)
One 100% whole-grain bun
   (for each burger)
Clean condiments for serving

1. Heat oil in a large nonstick skillet over medium-high heat.

2. In a large bowl, combine chicken, garlic, cumin, onion, mayonnaise, paprika, cheese, and salt and pepper to taste. Make sure all ingredients are evenly mixed.

3. Form two patties about ½-inch thick and place a small dimple with your thumb in the middle of each. Cook in the skillet over medium-high heat for about 6 minutes on each side, until cooked through.

4. Serve on a whole-grain bun with lettuce, tomato, and your choice of clean condiments.

EFFORTLESS KALE CHIPS

Going to the grocery store and buying kale chips is a complete waste of money. You only need a few ingredients and a little time to make your own for a fraction of the cost. Providing the crunch of a potato chip but healthier beyond comparison, these chips are easy to transport, inexpensive, and full of flavor.

1 to 2 bunches kale
1 tablespoon extra-virgin olive oil

½ teaspoon garlic powder
Salt

1. Preheat oven to 350 degrees.

2. Remove the stems from the kale and tear leaves into 2-inch pieces.

3. Wash and completely dry the kale leaves.

4. In a small bowl, mix oil, garlic powder, and salt to taste.

5. Toss kale leaves in the oil and spice mixture.

6. Line a noninsulated baking sheet with parchment paper and spread kale in a single layer, then place in oven.

7. Bake until crisp, 10 to 15 minutes, making sure not to burn them.

8. Serve warm or cold.

TURKEY MEATBALLS

Turkey is a wonderful substitute for red meat. Almost equally high in protein, but much leaner and with fewer calories per ounce, turkey's versatility allows it to work well in everything from lasagna to burgers. These meatballs are hearty enough to be eaten alone or with pasta.

Makes 20 meatballs

1 pound lean ground turkey
2 eggs, beaten
2 cloves garlic, minced
¼ cup finely chopped onion
¼ teaspoon salt

½ teaspoon black pepper
½ teaspoon dried oregano
½ cup dry 100% whole-wheat
   bread crumbs
1 teaspoon extra-virgin olive oil

1. Mix all ingredients except oil and shape into approximately twenty meatballs.

2. Coat a large nonstick skillet with oil.

3. Cook the meatballs for about 7 minutes, turning them to make sure they are browned evenly and cooked through.

GEORGIA PEACH SALMON

It's almost as if the culinary gods looked down on the earth and said, "Let there be peaches with your salmon." That's how divine the marriage is between these vastly different flavors. A recipe that is as simple as it is rich in flavor, you can whip this up in less than thirty minutes, but others will think it took you hours to perfect.

Serves 2

½ tablespoon grated fresh ginger
1 tablespoon rice vinegar
½ teaspoon fresh thyme leaves
2 tablespoons extra-virgin olive oil
¼ teaspoon salt
¼ teaspoon black pepper

1 tablespoon organic butter
1 teaspoon honey
½ teaspoon cinnamon
2 peaches, peeled and cut into
    wedges
Two 6-ounce salmon fillets

1. Preheat oven to 425 degrees.

2. In a small bowl, combine ginger, vinegar, thyme, 1 tablespoon oil, the salt, and pepper. Set aside.

3. In a small nonstick skillet, melt butter, stir in honey and cinnamon, then add peaches. Cook for 1 to 2 minutes, then flip the wedges and cook for another 1 to 2 minutes. Set aside.

4. Line a baking pan with foil and coat with the remaining tablespoon of oil. Season salmon with ginger mixture, then place on the foil-lined baking pan and bake for 5 minutes.

5. After 5 minutes, turn salmon over and coat with the peaches and sauce. Cook for another 5 minutes, or until flaky and the desired temperature is achieved.

6. Serve hot.

BAKED SWEET POTATO FRIES

Who says fries can't be healthy? This recipe should quickly remove all doubts. All of the nutritional power of the sweet potato is in its full glory underneath the crispy texture and robust flavors. Take the skin off or keep it on—either way, you can't go wrong. All you need is a few ingredients, a little bit of creativity, and fifteen minutes.

Serves 4

2 large sweet potatoes
Sea salt and freshly ground black
   pepper

2 tablespoons extra-virgin olive oil

1. Preheat oven to 425 degrees.

2. Peel the sweet potatoes, then cut them in half. Cut the halves into large slices, about ¾ inch thick. Cut these slices into fries at least ½ inch thick.

3. Arrange the fries on a baking sheet. Season with salt and pepper to taste, and drizzle with oil.

4. Bake for 15 to 20 minutes, until crispy. Serve hot.

DINNER

Lemon-Drizzled Grilled Chicken

Spicy Grilled Chicken

Grilled Chicken and Tomato-Lime Salsa

Seared Herbed Sea Bass

Oven-Baked Sea Bass

Sea Bass and Mango Salsa

Herb-Encrusted Grilled Tuna Steak

Deluxe Tuna Tartare

Cod with Zucchini Salsa

Turkey and Three Amigos Chili

Grilled Halibut with Tomatoes

Sweet Potato Pesto Pasta

Lemon Pasta with Chicken

Proteinaceous Salmon Pasta

Creole Salmon

Super Simple Herb-Encrusted Salmon

LEMON-DRIZZLED GRILLED CHICKEN

Sometimes the simplicity of a dish has an inverse relationship with the bigness of its taste. This is one of those situations—a little bit of lemon, salt, and pepper is all you need to dress up what would otherwise be a rather bland breast of chicken.

Serves 4

4 boneless, skinless chicken
   breasts
2½ tablespoons extra-virgin
   olive oil

1 lemon, halved
Kosher salt and freshly ground
   black pepper
⅓ cup fresh flat-leaf parsley

1. Preheat oven to 425 degrees.

2. Drizzle oil and squeezed lemon juice on chicken, then season with salt and pepper to taste. Place chicken breasts on broiler pan.

3. Cook for 4 minutes, then flip chicken and cook for another 3 minutes, or until cooked through. Flip breasts and continue cooking on high, 3 more minutes.

4. Remove chicken from oven, squeeze lemon juice on the breasts, and top with parsley.

SPICY GRILLED CHICKEN

A simple chicken dish that requires minimal ingredients and minimal preparation time is always welcome in the kitchen. If you like a little kick to your food, this is the recipe for you. This is not a dish that's going to cause flames to come from your ears, but it's just enough to get you to take an extra blink once you swallow it.

Serves 4

1 teaspoon garlic powder
1 teaspoon ground cumin
½ teaspoon ground coriander
3 tablespoons olive oil

½ teaspoon sea salt
¼ teaspoon black pepper
4 boneless, skinless chicken breasts

1. Preheat oven to 400 degrees.

2. In a small bowl, mix garlic powder, cumin, coriander, oil, salt, and pepper.

3. Use a basting brush to rub mixture over both sides of chicken.

4. Place chicken on a broiler pan and bake on each side for about 5 minutes, depending on the thickness of the breast. Make sure to cook all the way through so that there's no pink in the middle.

5. Serve hot.

GRILLED CHICKEN AND TOMATO-LIME SALSA

Chicken without seasoning is not the most exciting thing to eat. But when you throw on some tomato lime salsa, then you have an entirely different experience. The lime juice, scallions, tomatoes, and garlic provide a robust array of flavors that will leave you wanting more.

Serves 4

3 ripe tomatoes, diced
½ cup finely chopped fresh cilantro
2 cloves garlic, finely chopped
3 scallions (green parts), thinly
    sliced
3 tablespoons extra-virgin olive oil

2 tablespoons fresh lime juice
Finely grated zest of 1 lime
½ teaspoon sea salt
½ teaspoon black pepper
4 boneless, skinless chicken breasts

1. Preheat oven to 400 degrees.

2. In a medium bowl, make salsa: combine tomatoes, cilantro, garlic, scallions, 1 tablespoon oil, the lime juice, lime zest, ¼ teaspoon salt, and ¼ teaspoon pepper.

3. For the seasoning: In a second medium bowl, mix remaining oil, salt, and pepper.

4. Add chicken to the seasoning bowl and toss well.

5. Lay the chicken breasts on a broiler pan and place in the oven. Bake on each side for about 4 minutes, until cooked through and there's no pink in the middle.

6. Transfer chicken to a clean cutting surface and slice each breast diagonally to desired thickness.

7. Arrange chicken on serving platter and cover with salsa. Serve at desired temperature alone or over a bed of greens.

SEARED HERBED SEA BASS

A simple preparation with just a few ingredients delivers a fantastic sea bass. The relatively neutral taste of the fish allows the seasoning to work its magic without being overwhelming. It's difficult not to enjoy a dish this unassuming but oh-so-good.

Serves 2

1½ tablespoons extra-virgin olive oil

2 cloves garlic, chopped

¼ teaspoon onion powder

¼ teaspoon paprika

¼ teaspoon lemon pepper

Sea salt and freshly ground black pepper

Two 6-ounce sea bass fillets

1 tablespoon chopped fresh flat-leaf parsley

1. Put a large nonstick skillet over high heat and pour in 1 tablespoon oil. Add garlic and cook until golden brown, being careful not to burn it.

2. In a small bowl, stir together the garlic, onion powder, paprika, lemon pepper, salt, and black pepper to taste.

3. Rub the seasoning mixture evenly on both sides of fish.

4. Place fish in skillet, skinned side down, and hold down the edges so they don't curl for 1 minute, then turn the heat down to medium. Cook for 3 to 4 minutes.

5. Once skin is crisp and brown and the flesh is cooked at least two-thirds through, turn and cook on the fleshy side for a couple of minutes.

6. Sprinkle with parsley and serve hot.

OVEN-BAKED SEA BASS

After a long day, you might not be in the mood for a complicated, time-consuming meal. Sea bass is a perfect choice,
because with little work you can produce a flavorful fish that
is both light and filling (with 40 grams of protein) at the same
time. A few ingredients and a hot oven, and fish that's low in
calories but high in taste will soon be on your table.

Serves 2

2 cloves garlic, minced
1 tablespoon Italian seasoning
1 tablespoon extra-virgin olive oil
1 teaspoon chopped flat-leaf parsley
1 teaspoon black pepper

1 teaspoon sea salt
Two 6-ounce sea bass fillets
⅓ cup white wine vinegar
2 lemon wedges

1. Preheat oven to 450 degrees.

2. In a small bowl, mix garlic, Italian seasoning, oil, parsley, pepper, and salt.

3. Place fish in baking pan and rub mixture on both sides of fish
evenly, then pour vinegar over fish.

4. Bake for 10 to 15 minutes, until fish flakes.

5. Serve hot with lemon wedges.

SEA BASS AND MANGO SALSA

A sweet mango salsa is one of those dishes that can accessorize almost any entrée and make it taste better. The peppers and mango combine to give the preparation a satisfying sweetness with a little kick. This is a whimsical dish that's fun to serve.

Serves 4

2 tablespoons extra-virgin olive oil
¼ teaspoon pepper
¼ teaspoons sea salt
Four 6-ounce sea bass fillets
3 mangoes, diced

1 red bell pepper, diced
2 red onions, chopped
¼ cup finely chopped
   fresh cilantro
Juice of 1 lime

1. Preheat oven to 400 degrees.

2. In a small bowl, mix 1 tablespoon oil, the pepper, and salt. Brush the fish with the mixture on both sides equally.

3. Place fish in a glass or ceramic baking pan and bake for 5 to 7 minutes on each side, until opaque in the center.

4. In a large bowl, mix the mangoes, pepper, onions, cilantro, lime juice, and remaining olive oil.

5. Arrange the mango salsa on the fish and serve.

HERB-ENCRUSTED GRILLED TUNA STEAK

For the meat lover who wants to eat fish and the fish lover who misses the taste of meat, this tuna steak answers the call. It doesn't take a lot to deliver this neat package of smooth flavors. With only seven ingredients and less than thirty minutes, this recipe hits the mark.

Serves 4

2 tablespoons fresh lemon juice
2 cloves garlic, minced
1 tablespoon extra-virgin olive oil
½ teaspoon dried thyme

Four 6-ounce tuna steaks
¼ teaspoon salt
¼ teaspoon black pepper

1. Preheat oven to 400°F.

2. In a large glass bowl or baking pan, combine lemon juice, garlic, oil, and thyme. Add fish to the mixture and coat thoroughly. Cover and refrigerate for 20 minutes, turning after 10 minutes.

3. Remove tuna from bowl and season with salt and pepper.

4. Spray a baking pan before placing the tuna on it. Bake for 10 to 12 minutes, making sure you turn it over at the midpoint. Check the center to make sure it's the temperature you desire.

5. Serve hot.

DELUXE TUNA TARTARE

Not all fish tastes great raw, but fresh tuna is truly in a class by itself. One of the most popular sushi fish, it can be easily accessorized with seasonings and other ingredients that make it a light, refreshing treat. Feel free to play with the seasoning in this recipe to add other flavors that you might enjoy.

Makes 6–8 pieces

12 ounces sushi-grade fresh tuna, cut into ¼-inch dice

2 ripe plum tomatoes, seeded and chopped

1 small shallot, finely minced

12 fresh basil leaves, roughly chopped

1½ tablespoons extra-virgin olive oil

Juice of 1 lime

Sea salt and freshly ground black pepper

1 ripe Hass avocado, halved, peeled, and pitted

One 100% whole-grain or 100% whole-wheat baguette, sliced into thin rounds, toasted

1. Combine tuna, tomatoes, shallot, and basil in a large bowl and mix well.

2. In a separate bowl combine olive oil, lime juice, and salt and pepper to taste.

3. Add the oil mixture to the tuna mixture and mix well.

4. Add avocado to the tuna mixture.

5. Let mixture sit refrigerated for 1 hour to allow flavors to blend.

6. Serve slightly chilled, with baguette toasts.

COD WITH ZUCCHINI SALSA

This low-calorie, low-fat dish is high in flavor and heart-healthy nutrients. The salsa blends well with the native flavor of the fish in an exciting array of color. Easy to fix, wonderful to taste, this dish gives a new meaning to the wide possibilities of cod.

Serves 4

FOR THE SALSA:

1 tablespoon finely chopped fresh basil

1½ teaspoons capers, rinsed and drained

1 clove garlic, peeled and minced

2 teaspoons fresh lemon juice

2 teaspoons extra-virgin olive oil

1 tablespoon finely chopped fresh flat-leaf parsley

2 tablespoons finely chopped red onion

⅛ teaspoon black pepper

½ cup finely chopped roasted peppers

1½ cups chopped tomatoes

1½ cups chopped zucchini

FOR THE FISH:

Four 6-ounce cod fillets (with or without skin)

¼ teaspoon lemon pepper

1 tablespoon extra-virgin olive oil

FOR THE SALSA:

In a large bowl, combine all salsa ingredients and mix well to incorporate. Cover and refrigerate.

FOR THE FISH:

1. Pat the cod fillets dry and season with lemon pepper.

2. Heat oil in nonstick skillet over medium-high heat. Sauté fillets for 4 minutes on each side or until fish flakes with a fork. Do not overcook.

3. Serve hot with salsa spooned over top.

TURKEY AND THREE AMIGOS CHILI

Who says that beef has a monopoly on great chili? This dish utilizes the power of turkey's wonderful ability to absorb surrounding flavors. The team of three beans offers another punch of protein and a melding of textures and flavors that make this dish savory and filling.

Serves 6 to 8

2 tablespoons extra-virgin olive oil

1 pound lean ground turkey

1 yellow onion, chopped

3 cloves garlic, chopped

1 yellow bell pepper, chopped

1 tablespoon tomato paste or Tomato Puree (see recipe, page 198)

1 tablespoon chili powder

One 14-ounce can organic crushed tomatoes

2 cups water mixed with 2 tablespoons extra-virgin olive oil

One 15-ounce can reduced-sodium cannellini beans, rinsed and drained

One 15-ounce can reduced-sodium kidney beans, rinsed and drained

One 15-ounce can reduced-sodium pinto beans, rinsed and drained

Freshly ground black pepper and salt

Sliced scallions for serving

1. Heat oil in a large saucepan over medium heat. Add turkey and break it up with a wooden spoon. Cook until browned, 6 to 8 minutes. Add onion, garlic, and bell pepper and cook, stirring, until softened, 6 to 8 minutes.

2. Add tomato paste and chili powder and cook, stirring, until the paste begins to caramelize, 3 to 4 minutes.

3. Add water and oil mixture and bring to a simmer and cook until liquid has reduced by half, about 5 minutes. Add tomatoes, water with oil in it, and beans. Bring to a boil.

4. Reduce the heat to a simmer, cover, and cook until very thick, 35 to 40 minutes. Season with pepper and salt to taste. Garnish with the scallions and serve.

GRILLED HALIBUT WITH TOMATOES

Get ready to load up with the protein in this halibut dish that will take only minutes to prepare. The tomatoes and fresh juice add a spike of sweetness and mild acidity that give the mild-flavored fish a little edge and excitement.

Serves 4

2 tablespoons extra-virgin olive oil
2 cloves garlic, minced
½ cup fresh orange juice
¼ cup fresh flat-leaf parsley leaves
1 pint cherry tomatoes, cut in half

½ teaspoon sea salt
½ teaspoon black pepper
Four 6-ounce pieces skinless
    halibut fillet

1. In a large nonstick skillet, heat 1 tablespoon oil. Add garlic and cook, stirring often, until fragrant, about 30 seconds.

2. Add orange juice, parsley, tomatoes, ¼ teaspoon salt, and ¼ teaspoon pepper and simmer until tomatoes begin to break down, about 5 minutes.

3. Heat remaining oil in a large nonstick skillet over medium heat. Season fish with remaining salt and pepper. Cook about 5 minutes per side, until it flakes with a fork.

4. Serve with tomatoes on the side.

SWEET POTATO PESTO PASTA

This vegetarian pasta dish is cooked in the classic Genovese tradition with pesto, potatoes, and green beans. Easy to make, the flavors blend well together and the different textures of smooth and firm keep each bite interesting. In less than thirty minutes you'll have a tasty, nutrient-dense dish that may not be the classic pesto preparation, but one everyone can enjoy.

Serves 4

1 cup frozen shelled edamame, thawed

2 cloves garlic, chopped

¼ cup sliced almonds, toasted

¼ cup fresh flat-leaf parsley leaves

Grated zest of ½ lemon

½ cup freshly grated parmesan cheese, plus more for garnish

¼ cup extra-virgin olive oil, plus more as needed

Sea salt and freshly ground black pepper

1 pound whole-wheat spaghetti or penne pasta

2 sweet potatoes, cut into ¾-inch cubes

30 green beans, trimmed and cut in half

1. To make pesto sauce, combine edamame, garlic, and almonds in the bowl of a food processor and pulse until finely chopped. Add parsley, lemon zest, parmesan, and oil and pulse until well combined and the edamame is very finely chopped. Transfer pesto to a large mixing bowl and season with salt and pepper.

2. Bring a large pot of water to a boil with a pinch of salt, then boil pasta, sweet potatoes, and green beans until pasta is al dente and potato and green beans are very tender—about 10 minutes.

Drain, and reserve 4 tablespoons of the cooking water, setting it aside.

3. Transfer pasta, potatoes, and green beans to a large bowl. Stir in pesto and cooking water and toss well until the sauce is a creamy texture. Season with salt and pepper to taste. Divide among plates, drizzle with oil, and serve.

LEMON PASTA WITH CHICKEN

You can never go wrong with pasta and tender chunks of chicken. Add some lemon juice and you have a vibrant-flavored protein-packing dish that fills you up on relatively few calories with some whole grains as an added nutrient bonus.

Serves 4

1 pound whole-wheat penne pasta
Salt and freshly ground black
  pepper to taste
12 ounces raw, uncoated chicken
  tenders
2 tablespoons extra-virgin olive oil
2 cloves garlic, minced

8 cherry tomatoes, halved
¼ teaspoon red pepper flakes
Juice of 2 lemons
2 tablespoons roughly chopped
  fresh parsley
½ cup freshly grated parmesan
  cheese

1. Cook the pasta in a large pot of boiling salted water, until al dente. Drain well.

2. Season chicken with salt and pepper, then add 1 tablespoon of oil and chicken to a large skillet over medium-high heat. Cook until golden brown and cooked through. Remove from skillet and slice on a plate.

3. In a large saucepan, combine garlic, remaining oil, tomatoes, and red pepper flakes. Sauté chicken for 2 to 3 minutes, then add the cooked pasta. Cook for another 1 minute, then remove from the heat. Toss well with lemon juice. Pour all ingredients into a large bowl and mix again.

4. Serve garnished with parsley, with parmesan to sprinkle on top.

PROTEINACEOUS SALMON PASTA

The combination of pasta and salmon with a kick of lemon is difficult to resist. This simple recipe packs a powerful protein punch, with more than 30 grams per serving. Feel free to mix in your preferred vegetables to add some fiber and make the dish not only delicious but filling as well.

Serves 4

1 pound whole-wheat penne or rigatoni pasta
Sea salt and freshly ground black pepper
One 1-pound salmon fillet
½ cup fresh basil leaves, finely chopped
2 teaspoons capers, drained and rinsed
2 cloves garlic, minced
Grated zest and juice of 1 lemon
2 tablespoons extra-virgin olive oil
½ teaspoon red pepper flakes
About 1 teaspoon freshly grated Parmesan cheese

1. Preheat oven to 375 degrees.

2. Cook pasta in a large pot of boiling salted water, until al dente. Drain well.

3. Season salmon with salt and pepper to taste, then place on a parchment paper–lined baking pan and bake for 15 to 20 minutes, until desired temperature is reached.

4. In a large bowl, toss pasta with basil, capers, garlic, lemon zest, lemon juice, oil, red pepper flakes, and salt and pepper to taste.

5. Cut salmon into bite-size pieces. Add it to the pasta bowl and gently toss, making sure not to break up the salmon pieces.

6. Serve hot, topped with parmesan.

CREOLE SALMON

If you're looking for a little Cajun-style kick with your salmon, this recipe is all you need. The combination of Creole seasoning and Greek yogurt delivers a flavorful punch that will have you cleaning your plate. An easy dish to prepare, you can whip this up with a complement of green beans and be ready for a feast.

Serves 4

1 pound green beans, trimmed
1 teaspoon fresh lemon juice
1 tablespoon extra-virgin olive oil
¼ teaspoon salt
¼ teaspoon pepper
⅓ cup nonfat plain Greek yogurt

2 teaspoons Creole seasoning
1 teaspoon chili powder
1 teaspoon paprika
1 teaspoon grated lemon zest
Four 6-ounce salmon fillets
½ cup finely chopped toasted pecans

1. Preheat oven to 425 degrees.

2. Line a large baking pan with foil.

3. In a large bowl, toss green beans, lemon juice, oil, salt, and pepper, then arrange in pan and bake for 5 to 7 minutes.

4. In the same bowl, stir together yogurt, Creole seasoning, chili powder, paprika, and lemon zest. Spread onto four salmon fillets; top with pecans.

5. Move beans to outer edge of pan and place salmon fillets in the center.

6. Bake 10 minutes per 1 inch of thickness measured at thickest part of fillets.

7. Serve hot.

SUPER SIMPLE HERB-ENCRUSTED SALMON

It doesn't get much easier than this. The versatile nature of this fish allows you to create a flavorful dish with little effort and few ingredients. You can adjust the spice selection to something that better suits your taste buds. Use this recipe as a blueprint and have lots of fun.

Serves 4

1 tablespoon dried basil
1 teaspoon ground cumin
1 tablespoon garlic powder
½ teaspoon salt

2 tablespoons extra-virgin
  olive oil
4 six-ounce salmon fillets
4 lemon wedges

1. Stir together the basil, cumin, garlic powder, and salt in a small bowl, then rub onto the salmon fillets.

2. Pour the oil in a non-stick sauté pan over medium heat.

3. Cook the salmon until browned and flaky (test with a fork), about 5–6 minutes per side.

4. Serve each piece of salmon with a lemon wedge.

CONDIMENTS

Homemade Ketchup

Clean Mayonnaise

Orange Raspberry Vinaigrette

Honey Balsamic Vinaigrette

Quick Salsa Fresca

HOMEMADE KETCHUP

2 tablespoons extra-virgin olive oil
1 onion, diced
2 cloves garlic, minced
¼ teaspoon ground allspice
½ teaspoon chili powder
¼ teaspoon powdered ginger
½ teaspoon red pepper
   flakes
¼ cup apple cider vinegar
¼ cup organic honey

2 tablespoons organic tomato
   paste or Tomato Puree
   (see recipe, page 198)
One 28-ounce can peeled whole
   tomatoes in juice
1 tablespoon organic
   Worcestershire sauce
¼ teaspoon cinnamon
Salt and freshly ground black
   pepper

1. In a large saucepan, heat oil and onion over medium-high heat and sauté until translucent, about 8 minutes. Add garlic, allspice, chili powder, ginger, and red pepper flakes and cook for about 2 minutes.

2. Add vinegar, honey, tomato paste, tomatoes, Worcestershire sauce, cinnamon, and salt and pepper to taste, then cook for 3 minutes, stirring often. Bring to a slow boil, then lower to a simmer and use a spoon or spatula to crush the whole tomatoes and continue to simmer, uncovered, for 45 to 55 minutes, stirring occasionally, until very thick and smooth. Make sure to keep an eye on it and stir it to keep it from burning.

3. Chill in refrigerator for at least 1 hour to allow the ketchup to continue thickening and developing flavor.

CLEAN MAYONNAISE

1 large egg
1 egg yolk
½ teaspoon organic honey
1½ teaspoons fresh lemon juice
1 teaspoon organic mustard
2 teaspoons apple cider vinegar

½ teaspoon salt, plus more to taste
1 cup extra-virgin olive oil (this
makes the finished product a
little heavier, but we need to use
a clean ingredient)

IF USING A MIXING BOWL:

1. In a medium bowl, combine egg, egg yolk, honey, lemon juice, mustard, vinegar, and ½ teaspoon salt. Whisk until blended and thickened, 30 to 60 seconds. It should be a bright yellow.

2. In a very slow, steady stream, pour in ½ cup oil, whisking continuously, 3 to 5 minutes. Gradually add the remaining ½ cup, whisking continuously until mayonnaise is thickened, about 6 minutes. Now the mayonnaise will appear lighter in color. Season with more salt if needed. Place in an airtight container and keep refrigerated.

IF USING A BLENDER:

1. Put the egg, egg yolk, honey, lemon juice, mustard, vinegar, and ½ teaspoon salt in a blender. Turn on blender, then slowly pour the oil in through the lid a drop at a time, then pour in a small, slow stream. Blend until mixture thickens.

2. Taste and adjust your seasoning accordingly.

3. Refrigerate in an airtight container.

ORANGE RASPBERRY VINAIGRETTE

½ cup freshly squeezed orange juice

¼ cup organic raspberry white balsamic vinegar

⅛ cup extra-virgin olive oil

1 teaspoon chopped fresh cilantro leaves

Salt and freshly ground black pepper

In a small bowl, whisk together orange juice, vinegar, oil, and cilantro. Season with salt and pepper to taste.

HONEY BALSAMIC VINAIGRETTE

½ teaspoon minced fresh
   basil leaves
1 tablespoon organic honey
1 cup extra-virgin olive oil
¼ teaspoon dried oregano

½ teaspoon dried rosemary
⅓ cup white balsamic vinegar
Sea salt and freshly ground
   black pepper

In a small bowl, whisk together basil, honey, oil, oregano, rosemary, and vinegar. Season with salt and pepper to taste.

QUICK SALSA FRESCA

Nothing comes alive in your mouth like a fresh salsa powered by tomatoes, peppers, garlic, and cilantro. While salsa is a great pairing with chips, it also goes easily with chicken, fish, and pasta. Salsa recipes should be treated like a blueprint created in pencil. Erase whatever you want and add seasonings and vegetables that suit your taste!

Makes 2 to 3 cups

3 tablespoons finely chopped
　　red onion
2 small cloves garlic, minced
3 cups boiling water
3 large ripe tomatoes, peeled,
　　seeded, and chopped
2 chile peppers (mild or hot)

2 tablespoons minced fresh
　　cilantro (or flat-leaf parsley)
2 tablespoons fresh lime juice
Pinch of ground cumin
Pinch of dried oregano
3 tablespoons black beans
　　(optional)
Sea salt and freshly ground pepper

1. Place onion and garlic in a fine-mesh strainer; 1 cup at a time, pour boiling water over them, then let drain.

2. Once onion and garlic have cooled, combine in a medium bowl with the tomatoes, peppers, cilantro, lime juice, cumin, oregano, and beans (if using). Season with salt and black pepper to taste.

3. Refrigerate for 1 to 2 hours to let the flavors blend and settle. This can be refrigerated for up to 1 week. If the salsa is too hot, add more tomatoes to lower the temperature.

Note: Be careful handling the peppers. Wash your hands immediately after with soap and water and don't touch your face or eyes to avoid irritation.

eight

■ ■ ■ ■ ■ ■ ■ ■ ■ ■ ■ ■ ■

Clean Snacks

Snacking is important to any balanced eating program, especially when you are trying to be mindful of your calories and trying to avoid overindulging when it's time for full meals. The snacks listed below are suggestions. You can choose to eat from this list or other snacks that meet the clean guidelines. Remember, no artificial ingredients are allowed, as we are avoiding processed foods as much as possible. Are you expected to be perfect? Absolutely not. But should you be able to go twenty days and eat clean snacks 85% of the time? Absolutely yes. You know the structure of your daily meal plan, so plan ahead and make sure you have access to clean snacks during the day and at home. If you aren't hungry, then go ahead and skip the snack.

- 1 orange
- 1 apple with almond butter (1 tablespoon)

- Mashed avocado on 100% whole-wheat or 100% whole-grain toast
- 1 cup fresh cherries
- 8-ounce fresh fruit smoothie
- Hard-boiled egg with seasoning
- 1 cup kale chips
- 1 cup roasted chickpeas tossed with extra-virgin olive oil
- ⅓ cup organic, no-sugar-added trail mix
- ¼ cup unshelled pecans
- 15 walnuts
- 15 cashews
- 20 raw almonds
- ⅓ cup mashed avocado and 8 carrot sticks
- 15 unroasted peanuts
- ½ cup black bean dip and veggie sticks (carrots or celery)
- ¾ cup baked apple chips
- ½ cup banana slices and 1 tablespoon organic peanut butter
- 2 slices grilled pineapple
- Fresh fruit popsicle (made only from freshly squeezed juice and frozen in cubes)
- Small baked sweet potato
- Small garden salad
- 1 cup berries
- 1 sliced red pepper with hummus
- 10 to 12 baked sweet potato fries brushed with extra-virgin olive oil and sea salt
- 16 baby carrots
- 1 banana
- 10 cherry tomatoes with salt, pepper, and splash of vinaigrette

- ½ cup mushrooms marinated in extra-virgin olive oil, salt, and pepper
- 1 cup watermelon and red onion salad
- 8 watermelon and honeydew melon balls
- ½ cup raw veggies and pesto dip
- 3 cups plain air-popped popcorn
- 1 to 2 cups cucumber and tomato salad with extra-virgin olive oil, salt, and pepper to taste
- 15 frozen grapes
- ½ grapefruit
- 4 clean turkey meatballs (1-inch diameter)
- 3 ounces turkey slices and raw veggies
- ⅓ cup pumpkin seeds
- 1 cup mixed fruit salad
- 1 cup shelled edamame
- ½ cup cucumber slices and organic vinaigrette dressing
- 1 large beefsteak tomato slice and 1 tablespoon feta cheese
- ½ cup cottage cheese
- ⅔ cup raw veggies and guacamole
- 1 apple
- Ten 100% whole-grain pretzels
- ½ cup organic nonfat or low-fat cottage cheese
- Sliced tomatoes with a pinch of pepper and/or salt and olive oil
- 1 nonfat mozzarella cheese stick with a small apple
- ⅓ cup wasabi peas
- 8 green olives
- ⅓ cup sunflower seeds
- 6 ounces organic low-fat or nonfat yogurt with ⅓ cup sliced fruit

- ⅔ cup cauliflower with 2 tablespoons hummus
- 1 celery stalk with either 2 tablespoons hummus or 2 tablespoons organic peanut butter
- 1 medium apple with 1 tablespoon organic peanut butter
- ⅓ cup egg salad made with Clean Mayonnaise (see mayonnaise recipe, page 233)
- 7 olives stuffed with 1 tablespoon feta or blue cheese
- 40 raw unsalted pistachios
- 6 watermelon and cucumber skewers on toothpicks with one cube feta cheese on each skewer
- ¼ cup raw mixed nuts (unsalted)
- 20 grapes with 10 almonds or cashews
- 1½ cups sugar snap peas
- 1 large apple, sliced, sprinkled with cinnamon
- 2 sticks low-fat string cheese
- Frozen banana slices made from 1 medium or large banana
- Loaded pepper slices: 1 cup red bell pepper slices topped with ¼ cup warm black beans and 1 tablespoon guacamole
- 10 walnut halves and 1 sliced kiwi

nine

■ ■ ■ ■ ■ ■ ■ ■ ■ ■ ■ ■ ■ ■

Exercises

The exercise expectation of this program is only twenty minutes per day. The key is not the length of time you exercise, but the quality of time. When you make a moderately vigorous effort at your physical movement plan, you are definitely going to see results. The idea is that there is flexibility. You can break up the day's plan into two sessions, if you like. As you become more conditioned and build up your strength and endurance, you will be able to do it in one session. Below, find descriptions of some of the exercises that you can do to complete your physical activity for the assigned day. You can also do other exercises that aren't listed below, but try to focus on body weight exercises. If you have access to gym equipment, such as an elliptical, stationary bicycle, treadmill, row machine, and so on, feel free to incorporate them. The more you change up your workout with different exercises, the more productive and faster the results will be. Work hard and have *fun*!

Burpees

1. Stand with your feet spread hip-width apart and your arms resting down by your side. Put more of your weight on the front portion of your feet with your heels slightly off the ground.

2. Lower yourself into a squat position, making sure you steady yourself by placing your hands flat on the floor in front of you.

3. Once you reach the squat position and your hands are on the floor, quickly kick your legs backward so that your body is extended into a push-up position.

4. Lower your chest to an inch above the floor just as you would if doing a push-up. Make sure you don't let your chest hit the floor.

5. In one motion, push your chest back up and kick your legs forward so that you're back into a squat position.

6. From the squat position, use your legs to push off the ground and jump as high as you can into the air, then repeat from step 1 again.

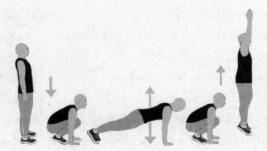

Exercise Variation: Plant your hands on an elevated platform about knee high—a bench or chair, anything that won't move. Take one foot and step back with it. Then take the other foot back until you are in a plank/push-up position. Hold this position for a second, then bring the first foot back forward. Next, bring the second foot forward. Once both feet are together, stand back up. Repeat the cycle. There is no push-up or jumping. Just the legs going back and forth and you standing.

Ice skaters

Think about the motion of competitive speed skaters as they move around the rink.

1. Start with your feet a little wider than your shoulders. Looking directly forward, keep your back straight and your knees slightly bent.

2. In one motion, take your right leg and extend it behind you toward the left side of your body so that it is further left than your left leg; take your left hand and bend it down toward the right side of your body and touch the ground.

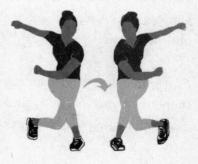

3. Next, do the same motion, but switch sides. Bring your right leg back to its starting position and at the same time bring your left leg across behind the right

side of your body; at the same time touch the ground in front of your left side with your right hand.

4. Repeat this alternating movement for the desired number of reps.

High knees

1. Stand straight with your feet apart no wider than your hips. Make sure your arms are hanging down by your sides and your back is straight as you look forward.

2. Jump from one foot to another as if running in place, making sure that you lift your knees as high as possible.

3. Your arms should be bent to ninety degrees with your hands clamped into a fist. Pump your arms up and down in the same motion as your legs.

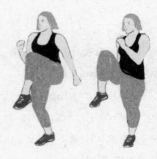

4. Be light on your feet; make sure your heels never strike the ground, but only the balls of your feet as you continue the jumping motion for the duration of the exercise.

Exercise Variation: If you are having difficulty with your balance, simply rest your hands against a wall and do the leg pumping motion, bringing your knees as high as possible.

Mountain climbers

1. Starting position: Start as if in a push-up position, but with your hands wider than your shoulders and in front. Slightly elevate your buttocks, but not too high. Start with your left foot forward until it comes to rest on the floor under your chest. At this point your left knee and hip are bent, and your thigh is in toward your chest. Your right knee should be off the ground, making your right leg extended straight and strong. Your right toes are tucked under, heel up. Contract your abdominal muscles to stabilize your spine.

2. Keep your hands firmly on the ground, and jump so that you can switch leg positions. Now your left leg is extended straight behind you and your right leg is bent underneath your chest with your right foot on the 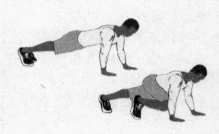 floor. Be sure to keep your abdominals engaged and shoulders strong. Do not lift your buttocks too high, as that will defeat the purpose of the exercise. Keep your head up and looking forward.

Exercise Variation: If you have a physical impairment that limits the range of motion in your hips, place your hands on a step or platform to get better leverage. Instead of shifting all your weight forward onto your front foot, keep your weight evenly distributed on both legs. Allow the step or platform to hold most of your weight so that there's less work for your legs to do.

Flights of steps

This exercise is simple. It is as it sounds—going up and down a flight of steps. Each flight should have between 10 and 15 steps. Going up and down a flight is considered to be one trip. So if the plan calls for 10 flights, that means going up and down 10 flights. You can do the flights consecutively, or you can break them up according to whatever works best for you.

Squats

1. Stand in front of a chair. Place your feet shoulder-width apart. Put your hands straight out in front of you, chest-high so that they are parallel to the ground.

2. Bend down as if you're sitting in the chair and stop 1 inch above the chair. Hold

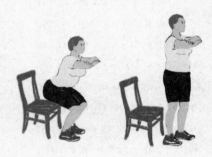

in that position for a 1-second count, then stand back up. Once you are fully erect, drop back into the next squat position.

Exercise Variation / **Wall squats**: Lower yourself into a squat position by pushing your hips back against a wall and keeping your heels flat and knees out. Keep your arms out in front of you parallel to the ground to help maintain balance. Hold the squat position for 5 seconds, then stand back up in an erect position. Repeat the cycle. As your strength improves, stay in the squat position for a longer time.

Steam Engines

1. Stand tall with your feet shoulder-width apart. Clasp your hands behind your head with elbows forward and in line with your shoulders.

2. Do these two things at the same time: raise your left knee up and bring your right elbow (hands still clasped behind your head) toward your knee, touching it if you can.

3. Once you complete this movement, bring your leg back down and your head back up. Then repeat the same movement with the opposite leg and arm (right knee up with left elbow touching it).

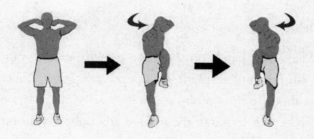

Exercise Variation: If you have physical limitations, you can still do this exercise. Instead of clasping your hands behind your head, put your arms in a 90-degree angle at your side with your hands balled into a fist and your forearms parallel to the ground. Take your right elbow across your body and at the same time lift your left knee. Try to touch your elbow to your knee or come as close as possible. Return to your original position and do the same on the opposite side.

Jog Punches

This is a simple exercise that is a variation of running in place. Stand in running position. As you begin to run in place, simply ball your hands into fists and punch them into the air, rapidly alternating them.

Exercise Variation: Instead of running in place, walk quickly in place and pump your arms in the air.

Plank

1. Plant your hands on the floor, directly under your shoulders, slightly wider than shoulder-width apart. Pretend that you're about to do a push-up.

2. Press your toes into the ground and tighten your butt muscles (glutes). Make sure you don't lock or hyperextend your knees.

3. Keep your head in line with your back, and neutralize the neck and spine by focusing on a spot on the floor.

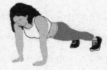

4. Hold this position for 15 seconds to start. The more comfortable and better conditioned you are, the longer you can hold the plank.

Exercise Variation / **Forearm Plank:**
Follow the same instructions as the regular plank, but set your forearms on the ground instead of your hands. Keep your palms flat on the ground in front of you or clasp them together—whichever is comfortable.

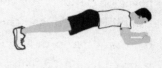

Exercise Variation / **Knee Plank:**
Rest your knees on the ground, with your forearms locked with your hands resting flat on the ground (the same position as for a regular plank). Having the knees on the ground reduces the stress in your lower back.

Marching Toward Bright Horizons

Now that your twenty-day journey is over, it doesn't mean that your health journey has come to an end. In many respects, you might be just starting the voyage that will engage and challenge you for the rest of your life. Hopefully, these twenty days have given you better insights into your strengths and weaknesses, your motivations, and your capacity to change, and an understanding of how much better you can feel and look when you fuel your body more efficiently and avoid the unhealthy sludge of processed foods.

Most important, keep a perspective that you are not and will never be perfect, but you *can* do better and *enjoy* the process. Establishing and maintaining balance in your life should always be a guiding force when making decisions or when you find yourself facing a difficult situation. Everything in life—including how you eat and move—has its place, and that place and its relationship to other aspects of your life must be respected. Happiness and being healthy are fraternal twins that make each other better. Feeling good internally and externally can be such a powerful motivator, validating the hard work and sacrifice that has led to your total transformation. If you can remember this as you navigate whatever lies ahead, you won't only measure your happiness in terms of pounds on a scale or calories in a cup; rather, you will measure it by how good you feel when you get up in the morning, your confidence to do whatever you want, and how much you laugh, not just at jokes, but at yourself as well.

index